Sleep
at
Last

Or How
Not To Be
An Insomniac

Paul James

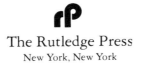

The Rutledge Press
New York, New York

· ·

.v blessings light on him that first invented this same sleep! It
.overs a man from top to toe, thoughts and all, like a cloak; it is
meat for the hungry, drink for the thirsty, heat for the cold, and
cold for the hot. It is the current coin that purchases all the
pleasures of the world cheap; and the balance that sets the king
and the shepherd, the fool and the wise man, even.

—*Cervantes 1547–1616*

· ·

Copyright © 1980 by Victorama Ltd.
Published by The Rutledge Press
A Division of W.H. Smith Publishers Inc.
112 Madison Avenue
New York, New York 10016
Manufactured in the United States of America
Edited by Sharyn Perlman
Designed by Allan Mogel
1 2 3 4 5 6 7 8 9 10
Library of Congress Cataloging in Publication Data

James, Paul.
    Sleep at last, or, How not be an insomniac.
    1. Insomnia. I. Title.

RC548.J35   616.8'49   81-15845
ISBN 0-8317-7419-3 (pbk.)   AACR2

Introduction

Man has been puzzling over sleep ever since he first woke up. Over twenty-five hundred years ago Homer decided that too much sleep was bad for you. More recently Shakespeare declared himself to be in favor of it:

> "Sleep that knits up the ravelled sleeve of care,
> The death of each day's life, sore labor's bath,
> Balm of hurt minds, great nature's second course,
> Chief nourisher in life's feast."

And only the other day Nietzsche pointed out that to sleep is no mean achievement: "To sleep at night we have to stay awake all day."

If we live to the age of ninety most of us will have spent a good thirty years in bed with our eyes shut, oblivious to all around us. Yet despite its importance, sleep is still one of the aspects of human life least understood by scientists and barely questioned by the human race at large.

To wit, some of the lesser-known facts about sleep:

• Complete lack of sleep will kill you more quickly than lack of food.

• The brain contains certain groups of cells which bring about sleep when stimulated.

• In a light sleep the body changes its position up to forty times in one night.

• There are two stages to our sleep: orthodox sleep when our bodies are completely relaxed, and paradoxical sleep when our bodies are active.

• Dreams occur during paradoxical sleep.

• We generally alternate between orthodox and paradoxical sleep at least five times a night.

• More time is spent in orthodox sleep than in paradoxical sleep.

• Twenty percent of our sleep is spent dreaming.

• The deepest sleep is in the early hours of the morning.

• Sleep is essential not only to rest the body, but to rest the brain.

• Lack of sleep will make a person irritable, irrational, and will eventually lead to mental derangement.

• Death occurs after ten days total lack of sleep.

• A newborn baby generally sleeps sixteen hours a day.

• On the average, people over sixty-five need only six hours sleep a night.

• The average person sleeps seven to eight hours a night, although needs vary individually as some people can exist on five while others need ten.

- Everybody dreams every night.
- Dreams are essential to good health and an active brain.
- Insomniacs may feel that they have not slept at all, but almost all sleep without realizing it.
- The major cause of insomnia is the fear that one will not be able to sleep.

All of this is very interesting as long as you're not reading it at three in the morning fretting that you've only got another four hours in bed before the daily grind starts again.

We know sleep is important and this book is dedicated to giving you a good night's rest. We want you to be able to sleep well, not just for tonight and tomorrow night, but for three hundred and sixty-five nights in a row—three hundred and sixty-six in leap years. If we're successful that should give you a cool two thousand nine hundred and twenty hours when you're dead to the world, or put another way, it will ensure that you spend one hundred and twenty-one days of next year without a care in the world.

Sounds great—but how does the book work? The answer's easy because *Sleep at Last* offers you two alternatives every night. Starting on January 1 and continuing until December 31 there's a different cure for insomnia for every night of the year, some physical, some mental, some demanding, some soothing, some uplifting, some exhausting—*all* of them well-tried and medically approved. No matter what may be keeping you awake, somewhere in this book there is a cure which you can repeat night after night once you've found it works.

If, despite the cures, you can't get to sleep immediately, don't worry. The book is also crammed with some fifteen hundred startling, amazing, bewildering, humorous, outrageous, outlandish, and bizarre items of factual information gathered together to entertain you during your lonely vigil until the soporific effects of the cures do carry you off to the land of dreams.

This is a book we want you to fall asleep while reading—and not many authors and publishers can say that.

Goodnight!

January 1

TONIGHT'S CURE

Autoslumber. Talk to each part of your anatomy separately telling each part to go to sleep. Start with your toes, then move on to the soles of your feet, then on to your ankles, your calves, your knees, your thighs, and so on until you reach the top of your head. Take your time, letting each limb relax slowly. By the time you reach your eyes you should be asleep.

TONIGHT'S TRIVIA

- The human brain is made up of 12 million cells.
- A safety pin was used in Greece in the eighth century B.C.
- Garlic belongs to the lily family.
- Man is the only animal that sleeps on its back.

January 2

TONIGHT'S CURE

Sinking. Concentrate on sinking through your mattress to the floor, then sink through the floor and continue downward. Simply lie on your back, close your eyes, and imagine that you are sinking down...down...down. Your body should feel really heavy. Don't worry about hitting the bottom—you'll be asleep by then!

TONIGHT'S TRIVIA

- Of all animals, the lion has the smallest heart.
- An ostrich egg has the same volume as two dozen hens' eggs. It takes forty minutes to boil, and one-and-a-half hours to hard boil. A man weighing 280 pounds could stand on the shell without breaking it.
- Buffalo Bill actually hunted bison.
- There has never been a U.S. president who was an only child.

January 3

TONIGHT'S CURE

Returning. In your imagination return to the house in which you were brought up as a child. Picture it from the outside, walk down the path toward the door. Once inside the house move systematically from room to room, taking note of *exactly* what is in each room. Your inspection of your childhood home must be as close and detailed as possible.

TONIGHT'S TRIVIA

- From the bottom of a well you can see stars even in daylight.
- What the English call a French letter the French call an English letter.
- The Turks called a turkey the American bird.
- Over half the time spent by U.S. courts of law is devoted to hearing cases involving automobiles.

January 4

TONIGHT'S CURE

Rotation. With your eyes open, rotate your eyeballs. While in the dark focus your eyes on the ceiling, then look to the right as far as you can, then down, then around to the left, then look back at the ceiling. Do this very fast, first to the right, then to the left. Close your eyes and repeat.

TONIGHT'S TRIVIA

- Tongue prints are as unique as finger prints.
- A full moon is nine times brighter than a half moon.
- A human neck has the same number of bones as a giraffe neck.
- Lemons contain more sugar than do strawberries.

January 5

TONIGHT'S CURE

Run wild. Imagine you are a beautiful wild animal—a horse, an antelope, a unicorn—and you are running across wide open plains, through lush green fields beside tranquil, soothing streams. Feel the warmth of the sunlight, the freshness of the air, the peace of your surroundings and fall into a deep slumber.

TONIGHT'S TRIVIA

- Frankfurter sausages were invented in China.
- Ants are capable of lifting fifty times their own weight and of pulling three hundred times their own weight.
- A hearse in Hartford, Connecticut, had the sinister registration number U2.
- George Handel composed a mass when he was just thirteen.

January 6

TONIGHT'S CURE

Out for the count. Lie back on your bed. Breathe in very deeply for a count of one. Hold it for a count of one. Breathe out for a count of one. Now breathe in very deeply and count one, two. Hold it, counting one, two. Release, counting one, two. Do this until you reach ten. If you have not dropped off by this time, repeat the exercise in reverse order from ten to one.

TONIGHT'S TRIVIA

- An elephant can carry over two gallons of water in its trunk.
- The Grand Inquisitor, Peter Arbuez, who had no fewer than forty thousand people burned at the stake, was made a saint by the Pope in 1860.
- The starfish has an eye on the end of each arm.
- The German poet, Hans von Thummel, was buried in the heart of an oak tree.

January 7

TONIGHT'S CURE

Heartbeat. Put your hand on your chest and feel your heart beating. If the room is very quiet you may even be able to hear your heart beat. Once you have traced the beat, start to count it. You will find that the constant rhythmical beat is both comforting and hypnotic.

TONIGHT'S TRIVIA

- There is no rice in rice paper. It is made from wood pulp.
- A flea can jump two hundred times its own length.
- Francis I, King of France in the sixteenth century, issued a decree making the wearing of whiskers punishable by death.
- Fireflies are so bright they can shine through the stomach of a frog that has eaten them.

January 8

TONIGHT'S CURE

Time change. Change your bedtime. Many people have a routine and go to bed regularly at the same time every night. If you have a set time for retiring to bed, but find it difficult to fall asleep once you are there, change your routine and go to bed at least two hours later. Don't waste the extra two hours watching TV. Use the time to catch up on those odd jobs around the house that you've been putting off.

TONIGHT'S TRIVIA

• A hippopotamus can run faster than a man.
• At the present time, there are approximately forty thousand direct descendants of Confucius (551–478 B.C.) living in China.
• Volleyball is the most popular sport played in American nudist camps.
• The largest eggs are laid by sharks.

January 9

TONIGHT'S CURE

Counting the hairs. The average scalp is said to contain one-hundred thousand hairs. Count the number of hairs on your own head, using your thumb and forefinger, and see if you compare with the average. It is easiest to begin at the crown of your head and work outwards. Whenever you lose count, start again from the beginning.

TONIGHT'S TRIVIA

• A red blood cell travels around the human body forty-three thousand times every month.
• The average person consumes approximately one ton of food and drink every year.
• The gestation period of a rhinocerous is 560 days.
• The most common name in the world is Muhammad.

January 10

TONIGHT'S CURE

Hot water bottle. Take a hot water bottle to bed with you. Place it against your stomach and lay the insides of your wrists against it. Blood flows around your body via your wrists and you will feel a glow of warmth that will relax you completely.

TONIGHT'S TRIVIA

• A bottle containing a message that drifted 1,250 miles across the Pacific in fifty-three days was found by a native who sadly could not read any of the eight languages in which the message was written.

• The French horn is neither French nor a horn. It is an English woodwind instrument.

• A fourteen-inch cube of gold weighs one ton.

• A scarf knitted from all the wool produced in Australia in one year could be wrapped around the world one hundred times.

January 11

TONIGHT'S CURE

Analysis. As you lie awake, analyze *why* you are awake. Are you too hot or too cold? Is there enough air in the room? Is there a noise that's disturbing you? Is your pillow lumpy? Are the blankets too light or too heavy? Decide precisely what is keeping you awake and then do something about it if you can or silently laugh about it if you can't.

TONIGHT'S TRIVIA

• Brushing your teeth with salt cleans them as effectively as brushing with toothpaste.

• The amount and type of food normally eaten by a human would kill a monkey in a very short time.

• The elephant is the only animal, excluding man, that can be taught to stand on its head.

• In certain parts of the world earrings are still considered an effective cure for sore eyes.

January 12

TONIGHT'S CURE

In a state. Name every state in the United States alphabetically. Then name the capital of each state, if you can. Finally, list each state you have lived in or visited and try to recall the year of your first visit.

TONIGHT'S TRIVIA

• If the Earth was composed of steel, it would weigh little more

than its scientifically computed weight—
6,552,000,000,000,000,000,000,000,000,000 (6 decillion and 552
nonillion) tons.

- The Dead Sea is so salty that it is impossible to drown in it unless you are held under the water.
- An elephant sleeps in a kneeling position.
- Barn owls consume more than their own weight in food every night.

January 13
. . . .

TONIGHT'S CURE

Black velvet. Close your eyes and imagine that they are covered with a piece of black velvet. Imagine that you are lying on black velvet, that the floors, walls, and ceiling of your room are covered completely in black velvet. Feel it, imagine the texture, and think about the *blackness*.

TONIGHT'S TRIVIA

- Oil and water *will* mix—if you add a little detergent.
- The oldest breed of dog is the greyhound, which was used for hunting by the Pharaohs in ancient Egypt.
- Peanuts are used in the manufacture of dynamite.
- In Jamaica there are oysters which live in trees.

January 14
. . . .

TONIGHT'S CURE

Bookworm. Before turning off the light, read a novel for at least half an hour, even if you feel sleepy before the time is up. After the half hour turn off the light and try to recall every detail of what you have just read. Remember the dialogues and how the situations were described, visualize the settings, work out what you think each of the characters looks like. Imagine yourself as the hero or heroine, and decide what you think will happen next.

TONIGHT'S TRIVIA

- Mosquitoes prefer to bite people with blonde hair.
- Queen bees lay as many as three thousand eggs in one day.
- Irving Berlin never learned to read or write music.
- Eighty-five percent of plant life on this planet is made up of greenery growing in the oceans.

January 15

TONIGHT'S CURE

Millionaire. Imagine that someone has just given you $1 million. Decide what would be the very first thing you would buy and who or what would be the first recipient of some of the money. Would you spend it all on one item, or would your purchase many smaller items? Work out exactly what you would do with every cent, for the only condition on which you can have the money is that you spend it all.

TONIGHT'S TRIVIA

• Clams can live for one hundred years.
• An alligator's bellow can be heard a mile away.
• It would take 2,487,996 years to rearrange 15 books into every possible combination, at the rate of one change per minute.
• After his first concert, Elvis Presley was advised to become a truck driver.

January 16

TONIGHT'S CURE

Problem page. Take some notepaper and a pencil to bed with you. Before turning off the light jot down absolutely everything that is on your mind at the moment: financial worries, emotional problems, family traumas, world crises, relationship upsets, career setbacks, and so on. Once you have written all this down, draw a line under it, turn off the light, and go to sleep.

TONIGHT'S TRIVIA

• The African elephant always sleeps standing up, which means that it is on its feet for over fifty years.
• Flies take off with a backward jump.
• Hungary is the largest exporter of hippopotamuses in Europe.
• Today was a dry day in the United States in 1920—Prohibition came into effect.

January 17

TONIGHT'S CURE

Attention! Before you get into bed stand smartly to attention beside it. Pretend you are a soldier. Imagine you are part of an honor guard on duty outside the White House. You must stand at attention until the President has walked past and inspected you. Stay in position, totally still, eyes straight in front of you, until your legs begin to ache and you start to feel drowsy. Remain erect and motionless until you just cannot stand any more—then all you have to do is fall into bed!

TONIGHT'S TRIVIA

- Emperor Nero tried to improve his voice by eating leeks.
- In 1887, in Montana, snowflakes fell that were eight inches thick and fifteen inches wide.
- In British Columbia it is illegal to ride camels on the road.
- Ostriches can swim, gorillas cannot.

January 18

TONIGHT'S CURE

Exercise. Spend today getting as much exercise as you can. Don't take a car if you can walk, use the stairs and not the elevator, and so on. Two hours before going to bed do some fairly strenuous physical exercise such as skipping or running in place, a few push-ups, or take a run around the block. If you use up all your excess energy during the day, by nightfall you'll be ready for bed.

TONIGHT'S TRIVIA

- The silkworm moth has eleven brains.
- X rays of the *Mona Lisa* reveal that Leonardo da Vinci painted three different versions of the same sitter.
- A few drops of black paint added to a can of white paint will make the latter whiter.
- Hummingbirds can fly backwards.

January 19

TONIGHT'S CURE

The lost hour. While elephants and dolphins can function with just two hours of sleep out of twenty-four, the average length of a night's sleep among human beings is now seven hours thirty-six minutes. Calculate how many hours you sleep each night and then make yourself sleep an hour *less*. The catch is that you must go to bed at the usual time—you lose the hour in the morning by getting up earlier than normal. After a week of this routine you will get into bed ready for sleep and insomnia will be no longer a problem.

TONIGHT'S TRIVIA

- The silk that spiders use to spin their webs is much stronger than steel thread of the same thickness.
- A cricket hears with its legs.
- It takes over ten years for a cork tree to grow one layer of cork.
- Bulls cannot distinguish red from any other color.

January 20

TONIGHT'S CURE

Flotation. Lie flat on your back. Close your eyes. Breathe in and out deeply for a couple of minutes, then allow your breathing to become gentle and relaxed. Now imagine your body is getting lighter and lighter and lighter until it has no weight at all. Feel the sensation of your body becoming so light that you float off the bed into the air. From there you float on, far away into the land of dreams.

TONIGHT'S TRIVIA

- Wolfgang Mozart's composition *Alleluia* consists of the title being sung over and over again. There are no other words.
- Attila the Hun is believed to have died of inebriation on his wedding night.
- King George I of England could not speak one word of English.
- Drumskins are often made from the parched skin of an ass.

January 21

TONIGHT'S CURE

Watch the birdie. Close your eyes. Imagine birds flying over your head. Picture them flying all around you. Think of a type of bird for each letter of the alphabet—albatross, buzzard, cuckoo, and so on. Once you have thought of twenty-six different birds, imagine each one in turn flying over you.

TONIGHT'S TRIVIA

- Man only has a use for about 4 percent of the plants on earth.
- The dangerous rays emanating from an atomic bomb disappear in a thousandth of a second.

- One of the most effective lobster baits is a brick soaked in paraffin.
- On January 21, 1824, General Thomas ("Stonewall") Jackson was born. A century later, to the day, Vladimir Lenin died.

January 22

TONIGHT'S CURE

Keep awake. Whatever happens, don't let yourself fall asleep! Tonight attempt to stay awake. Think about staying awake. Try as hard as you can to stay as wide awake as possible. Accept that you don't have to go to sleep and feel how good it is to lie in the dark and relax after a hard day's work, thinking your own thoughts, at peace with the world. When you really try to keep awake you will find it impossibly hard.

TONIGHT'S TRIVIA

- Figures as well as words can be palindromatic:

  $11^2 = 121$

  $111^2 = 12321$

  $1111^2 = 1234321$

  $11111^2 = 123454321$ and so on!
- A silkworm can consume eighty-six thousand times its own body weight in fifty-six days.
- There is a street in Canada that runs for a distance of nearly twelve hundred miles.
- Twenty percent of American families change residences every year.

January 23

TONIGHT'S CURE

Conjugation. Conjugate Latin verbs, or if you do not know Latin conjugate French, German, or even English verbs. Start with the present indicative active (amo, amas, amat, amamus, amatis, amant) and go right through the imperfect tense, the perfect tense, the pluperfect tense, not forgetting the future tense and the future-perfect tense. Always include the indicative passive as well as the indicative active and don't forget the subjunctive. When you have completed the regular and irregular verbs, move on to the declension of nouns.

TONIGHT'S TRIVIA

- Minus 40°C is the same as minus 40°F.
- In most countries more men than women commit suicide.
- One of the best ways of cleaning your teeth is by chewing a stick.
- We blink twenty-five times each minute.

January 24

TONIGHT'S CURE

Just strolling. If you are awake in the middle of the night, get out of bed and put on slippers and a robe. Do not turn on any lights, but stroll around your house or apartment in the dark visiting every room that is not occupied. When you return to bed, close your eyes and visualize each of the rooms you have just visited in as close detail as you can manage.

TONIGHT'S TRIVIA

- Not only did Anne Boleyn, second wife of King Henry VIII of England, have three breasts, she also had an extra finger on her left hand.
- A kiss is medically and correctly known as "The anatomical juxtaposition of two orbicularis oris muscles in a state of contraction."
- Cement becomes much stronger if sugar is added.
- Gold was discovered in California on January 24, 1848.

January 25

TONIGHT'S CURE

Comfort. One of the great problems when trying to fall asleep is finding a truly comfortable position. To appreciate real comfort, start by getting into the most *uncomfortable* position you can. Until you find it utterly unbearable lie face down with your arms folded behind your back and your face flat against the mattress. When you can no longer stand this, plump up your pillows and return to a normally comfortable pose. You will feel a whole lot better.

TONIGHT'S TRIVIA

- A clock loses weight as it unwinds.
- When women of importance died in ancient Egypt, cockle shells

full of cosmetics were buried with them to be used in the spirit world.

- In Istanbul there are nearly four-hundred fifty mosques.
- The American naval hero John Paul Jones ended his career by commanding the Russian Navy of Catherine the Great.

January 26

TONIGHT'S CURE

Snacks. Don't sleep on an empty stomach. Take a snack to bed with you. A New England tradition suggests that a quarter of an apple nibbled slowly before midnight ensures sound sleep after midnight. And the legendary Marlene Dietrich cured her insomnia by eating an onion and sardine sandwich before retiring. Whatever snack you choose try to avoid foods with a high sugar content—they may give you too much get-up-and-go.

TONIGHT'S TRIVIA

- The great actress Sarah Bernhardt played the role of the teenage Juliet in William Shakespeare's *Romeo and Juliet* when she was over seventy years old.
- Over thirty different shapes of unidentified flying objects have been spotted in the United States this century.
- It has been scientifically established that mice prefer women to men.
- Turkish baths did not originate in Turkey, but in Italy.

January 27

TONIGHT'S CURE

Senses. Try to imagine a series of situations in which you use each of your five senses in turn—taste, touch, sight, smell, and sound. First, imagine a favorite food or drink. Next imagine feeling something soft and gentle, like pure silk, a cat's fur, or the sun on your body. Then visualize something truly beautiful, an idyllic scene, or the girl or boy of your dreams. Sense the smell of wild flowers or exotic perfumes. Finally, listen to the sound of the sea.

TONIGHT'S TRIVIA

- There are more lakes in Canada than there are in the rest of the world.
- A prairie dog is not a dog but a rodent.

- Saudi Arabia imports camels from North Africa.
- You could fit the entire United States into Africa three and one-half times.

January 28

TONIGHT'S CURE

Numero uno. As you lie in bed start counting from one to infinity making sure you count in at least three different languages. Alternate the languages too, so that if you are using French, English, and German, your counting will go something like this: *Un,* two, *drei, quatre,* five, *sechs, sept,* eight, *neun, dix,* eleven, *zwölf,* etc.

TONIGHT'S TRIVIA

- In Australia there are eleven sheep to every human inhabitant.
- A horse has eighteen pairs of ribs.
- The whale is not a fish but a mammal and the female suckles its young.
- In the German state of Munster a plague of fleas was once formally banished.

January 29

TONIGHT'S CURE

Meditation. Put a candle or a nightlight in your bedroom. Place it in a dish of water so that if it happens to fall or burn down it will be extinguished and will not create a fire hazard. Place the burning candle so that you can see it clearly from your bed. Make sure all other lights are out and all you can see is this one flame. Gaze towards the flame, but not directly. Watch it dancing about. After a time you will get the sensation that the flame is growing. Feel the warmth and light being absorbed into your body. Let your thoughts wander, but keep your eyes on the flame.

TONIGHT'S TRIVIA

- A zebra is black with white stripes, not white with black stripes
- The last dodo died in 1681.
- A Sydney dentist grew a dwarf conifer tree in an extracted r
- W.C. Fields was born on January 29, 1897. During World
he kept $50,000 in a bank account in Hitler's Germany, "J
little bastard wins."

January 30

TONIGHT'S CURE

Recitation. What can you recite by heart: A poem of Edgar Allan Poe's, the Gettysburg Address, the Lord's Prayer, a song by Bob Dylan? Take the longest piece you know by heart and recite it to yourself. Once you have been through it forward and made no mistakes, recite it *backward.*

TONIGHT'S TRIVIA

- The Great Wall of China is one of the few man-made objects that can be seen from the moon.
- Marbles was played by the Romans as early as the first century A.D.
- An English scholar named Richard Porson (1750–1808) was able to recite all of John Milton's *Paradise Lost* backward as well as forward.
- On January 30, 1835, the first assassination attempt was made on a U.S. president. An assassin who thought he was King Richard III of England, and as such had a rightful claim to the United States, fired two handguns at Andrew Jackson. Neither went off and the assassin was confined to a lunatic asylum, where he outlived his intended victim by sixteen years.

January 31

TONIGHT'S CURE

Tick tock. Before you go to bed have a friend hide three clocks in your bedroom. They must be clocks that make a noise of some sort and your friend must on no account tell you where they are hidden. As you lie awake in the dark try to work out where each clock is hidden and try to guess which tick comes from which clock.

TONIGHT'S TRIVIA

- Dogs sweat through their paws.
- The Devil has appeared in more movies than Jesus Christ.
- Only the cock nightingale sings.
- Live toads and frogs have been found encased in stones, solid lumps of rock, and coal.

February 1

TONIGHT'S CURE

Heavy breathing. Lie on your back, eyes closed, mouth open, and relax. Now breathe in through your mouth very slowly, counting to ten. Hold your breath for a count of five, then breathe out through your nose counting to ten. Repeat breathing in through your nose and out through your mouth. Then in through the mouth and out through the nose continuing nose, mouth, mouth, nose. Keep breathing and keep counting.

TONIGHT'S TRIVIA

• There are 170,000,000,000,000,000,000,000,000,000 (170 nonillion) different ways to play the ten opening moves in a game of chess.
• The giant squid is the largest living animal without a backbone.
• A snake hears with its tongue.
• Clark Gable was born on February 1, 1907. At the height of his career, when he appeared bare beneath his shirt in *It Happened One Night*, sales of vests plummeted and a number of underwear manufacturers went out of business.

February 2

TONIGHT'S CURE

Bathtime. Before going to bed, have a warm herbal bath. Take four ounces of thyme and soak it in boiling water for ten minutes. Add this liquid to your bathwater and make sure that your bathwater is warm, but not hot. Fill the bath so most of your body is under water. Soak for fifteen to twenty minutes while letting your muscles relax and your cares drift away. Pat yourself dry with a big soft bath towel and get to bed as quickly as possible.

TONIGHT'S TRIVIA

• Giraffes show their love for each other by pressing their necks together.
• It takes forty years for vintage port to reach maturity.
• Queen Ranavalona of Madagascar prohibited her subjects from appearing in her dreams. If anyone did, he or she was put to deat'
• A Seattle man was recently charged with drunkenness. Not' strange about that, except his name was Al Cohol.

February 3

TONIGHT'S CURE

Insomnia. Take the word *insomnia* and as you lie awake compile a list of as many words as possible that can be formed from the eight letters. You should be able to get at least forty words, but remember you can only use the letters that are there and cannot use any of them twice. One and two letter words are acceptable, so you can use *I, a, in,* and so on.

TONIGHT'S TRIVIA

- The prehistoric dinosaur called stegosaurus weighed six and one-half tons but its brain weighed only two and one-half ounces.
- A kangaroo cannot jump with its tail off the ground.
- On the coast of Malaya there are clams large enough to devour a man.
- The tarantula spider cannot spin a web.

February 4

TONIGHT'S CURE

Cozy. Imagine you are a small animal—a puppy, a kitten, or even a baby—and tonight in your bed you are going to build the coziest nest imaginable. Put extra pillows around you so you have one on either side of you as well as one for your head. Curl up into a ball and pull the covers up as high as you can so you are as warm as possible. Lie there thinking to yourself, "How small and cozy and *secure* I am."

TONIGHT'S TRIVIA

- Gorillas are vegetarian—even the fiercest looking ones.
- One English prime minister used to sleep with each leg of his bed in a bowl of salt water to ward off evil spirits.
- Eskimos use refrigerators to keep their food from freezing.
- Catgut does not come from cats. It comes from sheep.

February 5

TONIGHT'S CURE

Think. Set your mind thinking about the great mysteries that have always puzzled you and to which there are no answers. For example, where did the universe come from? Surely there must have been a time when there was nothing. If God made the world then who made God? Imagine what life is like on other planets. Imagine what life must have been like on earth at the beginning of time. Imagine also what it will be like a million years from now.

TONIGHT'S TRIVIA

• Camel's hair brushes are not made from camel hair, but from squirrel's hair.
• One kilo of honey is a result of around one million bee journeys from flower to hive.
• A sharp cough will move air in the body faster than the speed of sound.
• The three-toed sloth is disguised by plants which actually grow on its body.

February 6

TONIGHT'S CURE

Still movement. Lie perfectly still on your back and close your eyes very tightly. Breathe gently, but positively. Imagine you are getting out of bed. In your mind, walk across the room to the door. Feel what it is like turning the handle. Make your way to the kitchen, taking careful note of every step. Imagine making a cup of tea or coffee. Get the cup, boil the kettle, fetch the milk, etc. When the drink is made, return to your room, remembering to close the door again. Imagine getting back into bed. You must make the whole journey in your mind without moving a single muscle.

TONIGHT'S TRIVIA

• In 1970 San Francisco's leading cabaret attraction was a "topless grandmother of eight."
• In 1896 there was a war between the United Kingdom and Zanzibar. It lasted thirty-eight minutes.
• James Madison, the fourth president of the United States, was only five feet six inches tall.
• On Philip Island, Australia, there is a natural rock formation that looks like an ice-cream cone.

February 7

TONIGHT'S CURE

Footbaths. Soaking your feet before retiring to bed could help you sleep. There are two methods. The first is to plunge your feet straight into a bowl of cold water and keep them there until the cold becomes unbearable. Dry your feet and get to bed as quickly as possible. If you find this too uncomfortable, have two bowls of water, one hot and one cold. Place your feet in the hot water and leave them there for a couple of minutes. Take your feet out and put them in the cold water for the same length of time. Return to the hot water. Repeat this five or six times. Just be sure to end with your feet in the cold bowl, and retire to bed immediately.

TONIGHT'S TRIVIA

• New York City originally had iron watch towers to spot fires.
• The water at the foot of Niagara Falls is warmer at the bottom than at the top. .
• Saturn has such a low density that it would float in water.
• The Beatles arrived in New York for the first time on February 7, 1964, when ten thousand screaming fans greeted them at Kennedy Airport. When the Beatles appeared on the *Ed Sullivan Show* it was reported that no major juvenile crime had been committed in the country during transmission.

February 8

TONIGHT'S CURE

Ear plugs. It may be a noise that is preventing you from getting to sleep. You may not have realized that the comforting tick tock of a bedside clock is in fact an irritant. Perhaps your sleeping partner snores or breathes heavily. Maybe that distant buzz of traffic is more disturbing that you imagined. If there is a possibility that noise is keeping you awake then ear plugs—available almost everywhere and usually costing no more than a dollar a pair—will be one of the best investments you ever made.

TONIGHT'S TRIVIA

• Until the fifteenth century diamonds were usually worn by men rather than women.
• A dragonfly can fold its legs into the shape of a basket to catch its prey.
• Buttermilk does not contain any butter as all the fat has been removed.
• A blue whale calf weighs ten tons at birth and reaches sexual maturity at the age of two and a half.

February 9

TONIGHT'S CURE

At the coast. Imagine you are beside the sea. Think of a resort that begins with the letter *S*. Now think of things connected with the seaside that begin with *S* such as sea, sand, surf, sky, swimming, skiing, etc. Name at least fifty things.

TONIGHT'S TRIVIA

- Mistletoe feeds off its own tree and will eventually kill it.
- The first pocket watch was made in 1510 by Peter Henlein.
- Sunlight does not penetrate beyond 444 yards into the sea.
- More than fifty thousand earthquakes take place on the earth every year, but many are so small they are not noticed.

February 10

TONIGHT'S CURE

Stretch. Lie back on your bed. Stretch each muscle as far as you can, then let it relax. Begin by extending your foot, toes downward, and stretch your toes as far apart as they will go. Relax. Push your heels toward the bottom of the bed and feel the stretch up your calves. Relax. Stretch your legs and thighs, pushing the backs of your knees downward. Relax. Squeeze the buttocks together really tightly. Relax. Continue for each and every muscle including your neck and shoulders. When you reach your head stretch your mouth into a really wide grin and then purse your lips. Relax. Move your scalp backward and forward. Screw your face up tightly and then relax. Your body should now feel heavy but good.

TONIGHT'S TRIVIA

- In 1975 a New Yorker was arrested for trying to drown his wife in a water bed.
- A ship called the *United States* crossed the Atlantic in 1952 in three days, ten hours, and forty minutes—the fastest crossing on record.
- Richard Wagner used to compose music wearing fancy dress.
- More than half of the world's silver is used in photography and the production of mirrors.

February 11

TONIGHT'S CURE

Shopping. Imagine you are shopping. Visualize a supermarket or store you generally visit. Buy one article for each letter of the alphabet, starting with *A*. If you are still not asleep by the time you reach zucchini, you must take your basket and return each item, remembering exactly what it is and where it belongs.

TONIGHT'S TRIVIA

• George Washington used to soak his dentures in port to improve their flavor.
• In 1909 a London barber shaved six men in one minute and then shaved a seventh man in twenty-seven seconds—blindfolded.
• In Switzerland the *soldanella* ("ice-flower") forces its way up through solid ice to blossom in the sun.
• Every year the Washington Monument sinks six inches.

February 12

TONIGHT'S CURE

Direction. Take a compass and see which direction your bed points. Find the North/South magnetic line and, if it is practical, move the bed so your head is pointing northward. Animals tend to be influenced by magnetism, especially birds who use magnetic forces for migration, and many people believe that humans are also affected by magnetism even though we cannot see or feel it.

TONIGHT'S TRIVIA

• People used to believe that cucumbers gave you cholera.
• Louis XIV of France took only three baths in his lifetime.
• Gioacchino Rossini composed most of his music while drunk.
• George Gershwin's *Rhapsody in Blue* was first performed on February 12, 1924, in New York's Aeolian Hall. Gershwin had been asked to compose the work for a special concert, but it wasn't until he read about it in the paper that he remembered and got to work—just in time!

February 13

TONIGHT'S CURE

Pooh, bah! Lie on your back and whisper the words *pooh* and *bah* to yourself while increasing their numbers. Always have one more pooh than bah. Begin with "pooh pooh bah," then whisper "pooh pooh pooh bah bah," then "pooh pooh pooh pooh bah bah bah" and so on. If at any time you lose track you must go back to "pooh pooh bah" and start the whole sequence over again.

TONIGHT'S TRIVIA

• The thirteenth day of a month is more likely to fall on a Friday than on any other day of the week.

• Research shows that more people transmit germs by shaking hands than by kissing.

• The platypus eats its own weight in worms every day.

• Enough water flows into the Atlantic Ocean from the Amazon River to supply two hundred times the municipal needs of the United States.

February 14

TONIGHT'S CURE

St. Valentine's. Do not sleep alone tonight. Find someone who is soft and warm and will hold you in their arms all night long. The warmth of someone beside you is comforting, reassuring, and relaxing—provided they do not snore. The feeling of protection and security with someone beside you is one of the best cures for insomnia. If you can't find anyone to sleep beside tonight, don't worry. *Imagining* someone works almost as well.

TONIGHT'S TRIVIA

• Pregnant women who smoke produce lighter babies than those who don't smoke.

• Edward Hughes once wrote four pages of notes on Jane Russell's bosom.

• In ancient times onions were considered an aphrodisiac.

• Oregon was granted statehood on February 14, 1859, and exactly fifty-three years later Arizona achieved its statehood.

February 15

TONIGHT'S CURE

School friends. Lie back, close your eyes, and think of a particular year in school or college. Remember the teachers or professors. Say the full names of each member of that class in alphabetical order, not just your particular friends, but everyone. Think of each person you are still in contact with. Imagine what each of the others is doing now, e.g., Mary Anne Honeyball will probably be married to a doctor and have four children, two boys and two girls; Cynthia Nelson will almost certainly be the president of the Oswego Gay Women's Workshop, etc.

TONIGHT'S TRIVIA

• James Knox Polk, the eleventh president of the United States, was unique. He fulfilled every one of his election promises.
• Leonardo da Vinci, painter of the *Mona Lisa*, was so strong he could bend iron bars with his hands.
• Molybdenum, a metal which has only been used in the manufacture of steel during the past fifty years, was known to the Romans thousands of years ago.
• There are at least 200 million left-handed people in the world.

February 16

TONIGHT'S CURE

Camphor pillow. The great Dutch artist, Vincent Van Gogh, cured his insomnia with a "strong dose" of camphor oil on his pillow. This is said to relieve any nasal congestion and, after a time, will safely dull your senses and ease you to sleep. Unfortunately, while the cure may help you sleep it won't automatically transform you into one of the greatest Postimpressionists.

TONIGHT'S TRIVIA

• The USSR, in 1920, was the first country to legalize abortion.
• In Cuba there is a crocodile farm where you can find as many as twelve thousand crocodiles at any one time.
• Half a dozen large fireflies will provide enough light for reading.
• A Hawaiian flower called the firecracker tree opens with a loud bang.

February 17

TONIGHT'S CURE

Onion intake. Take a large onion and cut it into rings. Take half of the rings and boil them for ten minutes in half a pint of water. Take the rest of the onions about one hour before retiring and eat them either on toast or in a sandwich. Add a spoonful of beef or vegetable broth mix or a stock cube to the onion water and drink it. This may not taste good but a lot of people swear it helps them fall asleep.

TONIGHT'S TRIVIA

- Sleeping babies are only six times less active than when they are awake.
- The state of Indonesia is made up of over thirteen thousand islands.
- The brain of Neanderthal man was bigger than modern man's brain.
- President James Garfield could simultaneously write Greek with one hand and Latin with the other.

February 18

TONIGHT'S CURE

Milky way. Lie in bed with your curtains open so you can see the sky very clearly. Look at the moon and the stars. See how many you can count. It has been said that if all the stars in the Milky Way were named it would take four thousand years to recite them all—and that is saying one name per second. While looking at the stars in the Milky Way start giving each one a name.

TONIGHT'S TRIVIA

- A holy man in Benares, India, named Hijmar held his left arm in the same position for over twelve years.
- Fingerprints have been used as a means of identification for 120 years.
- In the 1800s an unusual burglar alarm was invented. It was a door-lock that contained a small explosive that surprised a would-be thief with a loud bang.
- The owl cannot move its head from side to side.

February 19

TONIGHT'S CURE

Hyperventilation. Breathe in deeply and exhale fully. Breathe in again really deeply until your lungs feel as if they are going to burst, and exhale until your lungs are completely empty. Now breathe in deeply and hold your breath for as long as you can. Use your will power to resist the temptation to exhale and you will find that all thoughts are gone from your mind. When you can hold your breath no longer exhale slowly and with your breath will go all your tension. Now breathe in the beautiful cool air. Keep breathing steadily until you fall asleep.

TONIGHT'S TRIVIA

• India, although beset by famine, is the second largest producer of rice in the world.

• In Britain one person in ten plays the game of darts.

• Potato chips were invented by a Red Indian chef.

• Some of our body cells are so small that twenty thousand of them could fit on a pinhead.

February 20

TONIGHT'S CURE

Change of scenery. Rearrange the furniture in your bedroom, or if possible, move to another room. The insomniac becomes very familiar with how his or her bedroom looks in the dark and associates the shapes of things perceived with not being able to sleep. Rearranging the furniture gives the room an entirely new feel and may be more conducive to sleep.

TONIGHT'S TRIVIA

• From Mt. Irazo in Costa Rica it is possible to see both the Atlantic and Pacific Oceans.

• Lionesses at many zoos have been put on birth control pills.

• A lead weight and a leaf dropped in a vacuum will both land at the same time.

• On February 20, 1917, the United States bought the Dutch West Indies and on the same date forty-five years later John Glenn became the first American to enter the earth's orbit.

February 21

TONIGHT'S CURE

Vacation. As you lie in bed relive your favorite summer vacation. Imagine the hotel, the scenery, the sun, the sand, the sea, the places you visited, the people you saw, the foods you ate, and even the drinks you enjoyed. Recapture that feeling of relaxation and enjoyment. Feel the rejuvenating and healing warmth of the sun on your body and drift away into paradise.

- There is only one king termite and one queen termite in a termite nest. The other millions are their children.
- Panama hats are not made in Panama but in Colombia and Peru.
- The Romans used concrete.
- Only female mosquitoes bite people. The males are vegetarians.

February 22

· ·

TONIGHT'S CURE

Peppermint. Peppermint aids in inducing sleep. Either take a few drops of peppermint extract in a glass of warm water or suck a couple of peppermint candies and drink a glass of warm water just before you go to bed.

TONIGHT'S TRIVIA

- The tomato used to be considered poisonous.
- The average person is estimated to walk sixty-five thousand miles in a lifetime.
- The Chinese do not have slanted eyes—their eyelids are almond shaped.
- George Washington was born on February 22, 1732, but two other notable events took place on this date too. On February 22, 1819, Spain ceded Florida to the United States and sixty years later Frank Winfield Woolworth opened his first Woolworth's department store at Utica, New York.

February 23

· ·

TONIGHT'S CURE

Lullaby. Be lulled to sleep tonight with some sweet, soft sounds. Take a radio or cassette player to bed with you and play some of your favorite music. Don't have it on too loud (especially if you are not alone) and don't worry about the music continuing after you have fallen asleep. A cassette player is preferred to a radio because there are no commercials and the machine will automatically switch off when the tape ends.

TONIGHT'S TRIVIA

- The so-called impregnable Rock of Gibraltar is actually composed of soft limestone.
- The chalk used on a blackboard is made from plaster of paris.

- Baboons are capable of fighting and killing a fully grown leopard.
- At their closest points the USSR and the United States are just over two miles apart.

February 24

TONIGHT'S CURE

Stark staring. Lie back on your bed with the light out. Open your eyes and through the dark try to make out a particular object on the other side of the room. This can be an item of clothing, a door, a cupboard, or even a chair. Focus on this object and keep your eyes firmly on it without blinking. Remain like this for as long as you can, resisting all temptation to blink. Your eyes will start to feel heavy and tired but don't blink until you really cannot hold the position any longer.

TONIGHT'S TRIVIA

- Castration is the only known method of preventing baldness.
- A barn owl can see at night one hundred times better than a human being.
- Red squirrels attract more fleas than any other animal.
- Horses can sleep standing up.

February 25

TONIGHT'S CURE

Psalms. The most soothing of all psalms is *Psalm 23*. If you recite this to yourself very softly it will soon lull you to sleep.

The Lord is my shepherd; I shall not want.
He maketh me to lie down in green pastures:
He leadeth me beside the still waters.
He restoreth my soul: he leadeth me in the
paths of righteousness for his name's sake.
Yea, though I walk through the valley of the
shadow of death, I will fear no evil; for thou
art with me; thy rod and thy staff they comfort me.

TONIGHT'S TRIVIA

- The Holy Roman Empire was neither holy nor Roman—it was German.

- The sun burns an estimated 22-million billion (22 quadrillion) tons of hydrogen every year.
- The first railroads in the United States had wooden tracks.
- Camel's hair brushes were invented by a Mr. Camel. They contain no camel hair at all.

February 26

TONIGHT'S CURE

Drive on. Imagine that you are át the wheel of your automobile driving down a straight clear highway at night. All you can see is the road ahead. Very few people attempting this cure can "drive" for more than a mile without dropping off.

TONIGHT'S TRIVIA

- Napoleon's private surgeon could amputate a man's leg in fourteen seconds.
- The orange is one of the few fruits that will not ripen after plucking.
- The world's smallest church is in Covington, Kentucky. It seats three people.
- The Hawaiian alphabet has only twelve letters.

February 27

TONIGHT'S CURE

Tunneling. Close your eyes and think about the darkness behind your eyelids. "Look" at it. Experience the sensation of being in a tunnel and picture a small ray of light in the top right hand corner of the darkness. Imagine you are moving through this tunnel and continue until you are out in the open.

TONIGHT'S TRIVIA

- Queen Victoria of England wore a new pair of bloomers every day.
- The Romans ate doormice.
- An owl is the only bird that can look at an object with both eyes at the same time.
- Alphonse Duhamel built a clock out of an old bicycle.

February 28

TONIGHT'S CURE

Death bed. Imagine you are a superstar actor or actress performing a very dramatic role in a play. Imagine you are lovesick, stricken with grief, and on your death bed. Go through the last scene in the play gasping fond farewells to the love of your life who is at your bedside. The scene climaxes when you die five minutes before the final curtain falls. Once you have "died" you must remain motionless until the end of the scene.

TONIGHT'S TRIVIA

• An ostrich does not bury its head in the sand when frightened, only when covering its eggs or searching for food.
• Lions leave 90 percent of the killing of prey to the lionesses and then come along and eat the "lion's share."
• Early man dug graves from the shoulder blades of dinosaurs.
• In Italy thirteen is a lucky number.

February 29

TONIGHT'S CURE

Leap Year. This day occurs only once every four years which means that the age of people born on February 29 is a lot lower than anyone else's. Count how many leap years there have been in your lifetime and remember exactly what you were doing on February 29 last leap year. Assuming that you will live until you are 105, calculate how many more leap years there will be in your life span.

TONIGHT'S TRIVIA

• Man catches thirty different diseases from the common house fly.
• In 1957 the first American satellite launched at Cape Canaveral exploded only a few feet from the ground.
• It is said that a man of sixty-five is as strong as a twenty-five-year-old woman.
• Shredded wheat was the first breakfast cereal, produced in 1893.

March 1

TONIGHT'S CURE

Sheep counting. This is one of the oldest but still most effective cures. Visualize a five-bar gate. Concentrate on that gate and count the sheep that are jumping over it. Do not worry about where the sheep are coming from or where they are headed, simply count them as they jump over the gate. It is even harder to try and visualize the sheep jumping backward over the gate like a film shown in reverse.

TONIGHT'S TRIVIA

- Gale warnings were first issued in 1861.
- The Roman Emperor Caligula made his horse a consul.
- Leonardo Da Vinci could write with one hand while drawing with the other.
- Ludwig Beethoven composed most of his music after he had become stone deaf.

March 2

TONIGHT'S CURE

All at sea. Imagine you are lying on an air mattress in the middle of the ocean. (If you have a water bed this is quite easy.) Feel the gentle rocking of the water as you float across the waves. Feel the sun on your body and hear the sound of the waves. Imagine you will be floating here for the rest of time.

TONIGHT'S TRIVIA

- Rome and Madrid lie exactly due east of Chicago.
- In India 845 different dialects are spoken.
- Almost five hundred years ago Shakespeare mentioned America in his play *The Comedy of Errors*, act 3 scene 2.
- According to a newspaper poll in 1926 the most popular movie star was the dog Rin Tin Tin.

March 3

TONIGHT'S CURE

Milk. Before going to bed take a drink of hot milk. Heat the milk and then *either* sprinkle some nutmeg on it *or* add a teaspoon of honey, *or* malt *or* two teaspoons of black molasses. Drink the milk slowly and you should find it a soothing sedative.

TONIGHT'S TRIVIA

- Until this century natives of the Solomon Islands used dog teeth for currency.

- In Chinese script the character for the word *malice* depicts three women.
- Early blood transfusions used animal blood.
- The *Star Spangled Banner* was adopted by Congress as the National Anthem on March 3, 1931.

March 4

· ·

TONIGHT'S CURE

Back to school. They say that school days are the happiest days of your life. If your school days were happy, return in your mind to your school or college. Imagine the building from the outside. Enter the door through which you used to enter daily. Picture the stairs and the rooms one by one. Note exactly what is on the walls. Walk systematically around the building to the place that was always your favorite spot.

TONIGHT'S TRIVIA

- The oldest industry in New York is the fur trade, dating back to 1615.
- There is no lead in a lead pencil—it is graphite.
- The Greek philosopher, Aristotle, believed that the greatest delicacy was camel meat.
- The famous English naval captain, Horatio Nelson, suffered from sea sickness.

March 5

· ·

TONIGHT'S CURE

Around the block. Go for a walk around the block—literally—if it's warm enough and safe enough. If it isn't then get into bed and go for the walk in your mind. Picture every part of the walk, including every store or tree or parked car that you pass, as well as every individual you meet. When you get back home, take a hot shower in your mind as well.

TONIGHT'S TRIVIA

- In South Africa ostrich races are held with riders on each ostrich.
- One hundred and twenty drops of water are needed to fill a teaspoon.
- The female mosquito can produce 150,000,000,000 (150 trillion) offspring in one year.

• The largest shadow on earth is that of the moon during a lunar eclipse.

March 6

TONIGHT'S CURE

Wendy's age. In your head (or with a pencil and paper if you must) work out Wendy's age before you go to sleep. Wendy has three children under ten years old. The two oldest are twins. If the children's ages are written down in order, starting with the youngest, a three-digit number is obtained. Wendy's age is exactly divisible into this three-digit figure and the dividend is the sum of her children's ages. She is not a teenager. How old is Wendy?*

TONIGHT'S TRIVIA

• The first farmer's almanac was compiled in 1700 B.C.
• An anagram of astronomers is moon starers.
• The Cambodian alphabet has seventy-two letters.
• In the history of the world there have been ten years of war to every year of peace.

*Solution:

$$\frac{588}{5+8+8} = 28$$

Wendy is 28.

March 7

TONIGHT'S CURE

Neck rotation. Sit up in bed with your spine perfectly straight. Lean your head forward so your chin rests on your chest. Slowly rotate your head toward the right, so your right ear brushes past your right shoulder, and around until your head is as far back as it will go. Continue on to the left so your left ear brushes your left shoulder and around to the front to your original starting position. Your head has now gone full circle. Repeat twice more to the right and then rotate to the left. Feel the massaging effect this has and the way it releases the tension in your neck muscles.

TONIGHT'S TRIVIA

• Beethoven composed three sonatas when he was thirteen.

- There are eight cities called Rome in the United States.
- *Cha* is the Chinese name for tea.
- The center of the earth is four thousand miles beneath our feet.

March 8

TONIGHT'S CURE

House building. Tonight you can design and build the house of your dreams. First, in your mind's eye, picture the location. Then move through the house room by room picturing how you'd decorate and furnish each one. If you're still awake when you've completed the house, start laying out the surrounding grounds.

TONIGHT'S TRIVIA

- Until 1957 London was the largest city in the world.
- In 1890 red rain fell in Newfoundland.
- No matter what offences a Hindu man may commit he cannot be excommunicated.
- In the days when top hats were commonplace many doctors carried their stethoscopes under their hats.

March 9

TONIGHT'S CURE

Midnight feast. If every mental cure for insomnia has failed, get up. Don't put on your robe or slippers though. Go to the kitchen just as you are and cut yourself a thick slice of bread, preferably homemade, and chew each mouthful at least twenty times. When you finish, drink a glass of ice-cold milk. This will make you feel very cool and your feet may be quite cold. Hurry back to your bed and fall asleep in the welcoming warmth and comfort.

TONIGHT'S TRIVIA

- The Chenchu tribe in India believe that nighttime produces blind children.
- One-hundred eighty medical journals are published every hour around the world.
- Peanuts are not nuts, they are beans.
- Until 1973 no rain had fallen in Desierto de Atacama, Chile, for over four hundred years.

March 10

TONIGHT'S CURE

Agenda. If you're prone to insomnia always keep a pencil and note pad beside your bed. Then instead of uselessly lying awake in the dark write down what you have to do tomorrow, listing the most important things first. You'll find this will not only alleviate your worries about tomorrow, but it will also give you a clear routine for the day. Repeat the exercise tomorrow night but first check off all the things you have accomplished. It will be very reassuring to see what you have achieved, so reassuring you might fall asleep on its strength.

TONIGHT'S TRIVIA

- Over 70 percent of the earth is covered by sea.
- Fred Astaire's legs were insured for $650,000.
- Diamond is the hardest substance known to man.
- The shortest will on record (1895): "All to Mother."

March 11

TONIGHT'S CURE

Side sleep. Each of us finds it more comfortable to sleep on one side of our body than on the other. To begin this cure lie on your most comfortable side. Keep your lower leg straight and draw the knee of your other leg upward. Stretch the arm you're lying on outward across the bed and let the other arm hang in front of you, loose and relaxed. Let yourself relax completely and drift off to sleep.

TONIGHT'S TRIVIA

- The twenty-six letters of the English alphabet can be arranged into more than 29,000 quatrillion combinations.
- Ovid once wrote a book about cosmetics.
- The brassiere was first patented in 1914 by an American debutante named Caresse Crosby.
- In 1836 New York's Astor House hotel opened its doors to patrons for the first time and offered them a unique facility—hot, running water on the first floor.

March 12

TONIGHT'S CURE

Eight plus eight plus eight. Lie on your back and *without using your fingers or toes* start to count slowly in eights: eight, sixteen, twenty-four, thirty-two, forty, and so on. Continue adding eight in this way until you reach one thousand. If at any time you lose count, however, you have to go back to the beginning and start again with eight.

TONIGHT'S TRIVIA

• The eye of a fly has over four thousand facets enabling it to see an approaching enemy from every direction.
• The male spider's penis is on the end of one of its legs.
• A young hawk is called an eyas.
• Two important U.S. institutions came into being on March 12: In 1789 the U.S. Post Office was established, and in 1912 the Girl Scouts movement started.

March 13

TONIGHT'S CURE

Radio sleep. If you're the sort of person who tunes out when there's a murmur of voices you can't understand try turning your radio to a station that only broadcasts chat shows. Turn the volume down so the voices are muffled and it is impossible to hear what is actually being said. You will soon find yourself becoming bored with the sound and you'll drop off to sleep, just as many people do while watching TV.

TONIGHT'S TRIVIA

• The average lead pencil will draw a line thirty-five miles long.
• The sailfish can swim faster than a horse can gallop.
• The eggs of a kiwi are a quarter of its body weight.
• Clean snow takes longer to melt than dirty snow.

March 14

TONIGHT'S CURE

Darkness. Check how dark your room is tonight. It could be that a ray of light is keeping you awake. Pin a blanket up over the window so no light can penetrate. Stuff newspaper under the door to stop any light from shining underneath. Cover your luminous watch or alarm clock with a handkerchief. Black out the room completely and you'll soon fall asleep undisturbed in the total darkness.

TONIGHT'S TRIVIA

• In Argentina the "man in the moon" appears upside down.
• St. Luke was the only non-Jewish author of the New Testament.
• Japanese cherry trees bear no fruit.
• There is no soda in soda water.

March 15

TONIGHT'S CURE

Baby slumber. Do you remember what it felt like when you were a baby? Do you remember how you used to fall asleep in your carriage on warm afternoons? Even if that's all far behind you, you've still seen enough babies wrapped in cozy blankets, peacefully sleeping, to imagine how it must feel. So snuggle into your bed, curl up like a baby, and pretend that you're being gently rocked to sleep.

TONIGHT'S TRIVIA

• Flies prefer to breed in the center of a room.
• The Milan cathedral took 579 years to build.
• One ton of coal is needed to make one ton of paper.
• About one million meteors reach our atmosphere every hour.

March 16

TONIGHT'S CURE

Vinegar. If you can't sleep at night because you're always too hot and uncomfortable, take a bowl of vinegar and a wad of cotton. Soak the cotton in the vinegar and then gently dab your face. Once your face feels cool and fresh place the pad across your nose and inhale. Breathe in until the insides of the nostrils begin to prickle. Then lie back, as still as you can, and fall asleep.

TONIGHT'S TRIVIA

• The yo-yo was originally a Filipino jungle weapon.
• In 1863 twelve hundred people were killed in anti-conscription riots in New York.

- In 1976 a bottle of Chateau Lafite Rothschild was sold for $14,200.
- West Point was established on March 16, 1802. On the same day 181 years earlier the Pilgrim Fathers were visited by their first Indian who walked into camp and asked, in English, if he could have a beer.

March 17

TONIGHT'S CURE

Bathtime. Before going to bed fill the tub with cold water and plunge straight in for at least three minutes. If you cannot cope with the idea of a completely cold bath then add just enough hot water to make it lukewarm. You can also take a cold shower. Either way, pat yourself dry with a large soft bath towel. Do not rub yourself dry as this will only act as a stimulant and keep you awake. Then get to bed as quickly as possible and drift off to sleep.

TONIGHT'S TRIVIA

- In 1790 George Washington spent $200 in two months on ice cream.
- Up until 1859 baseball umpires used to sit in padded rocking chairs behind the catchers.
- An albatross is capable of flying without once flapping its wings.
- All Buddhists celebrate their birthday on New Year's Day.

March 18

TONIGHT'S CURE

Letter writing. Here's another use for the pad and pen you should always have near your bed if you suffer from insomnia. Catch up on that avalanche of correspondence that's kept you awake so many nights. Why not fill those wide-awake hours by answering your outstanding letters to friends? The house is quiet, you can think and write undisturbed, and for once you can concentrate completely on the letter. Don't answer business letters though—keep them for your working hours. This letter writing's for fun.

TONIGHT'S TRIVIA

- The late John Wayne was christened Marion Morrison.
- No two zebras have identical stripes.

- One quarter of the world's cattle live in India.
- Seedless oranges were not grown in the United States until 1871. The first ones were imported from Brazil and were planted in California.

March 19

TONIGHT'S CURE

Sleep. Lie on you back, or on your side if that is more comfortable. Close your eyes and say the word *sleep* to yourself. Don't say any other word. Close your mind to everything else and just say "sleep" over and over again. Picture the word in your mind. Picture the five letters and continue saying the word until you feel your eyelids growing heavier and heavier. Say "sleep" slowly, quickly, and with a one-beat pause in between. Say it in as many ways as you can and you'll exhaust yourself with all the possibilities.

TONIGHT'S TRIVIA

- Shirley Temple made over one million dollars before she was ten.
- If you lived in Shanghai and dug deep enough through the earth you would come out at Buenos Aires.
- An average person has a vocabulary of three thousand words.
- The front lawn of the White House was turned into a pasture during World War I—Woodrow Wilson's wife grazed sheep there.

March 20

TONIGHT'S CURE

Train journey. Imagine you are riding on a train to the destination of your dreams. Lie back in your seat. Feel the gentle rocking of the train. Gaze at the breathtaking scenery through the window as it flashes past. Picture the other passengers in the compartment. Perhaps they are friends or relatives who you would like to have along. Perhaps you are happy because they're not with you. Imagine the exotic smells drifting in from the open window and down the corridor. Close your eyes now and let the motion of the train rock you to sleep.

TONIGHT'S TRIVIA

- The breath of the billy goat was once thought to have healing powers.

- The fifth century King of Persia, Cyrus the Great, knew the name of every soldier in his army.
- Eunuchs do not suffer from adolescent acne.
- More snow falls in the Grand Canyon than in Minneapolis, Minnesota.

March 21

TONIGHT'S CURE

Tiny tot. Why not try a soothing nightcap to send you to sleep? Boil some milk in a saucepan and pour this into a cup or heatproof glass. Now add a small tot of liquor—whisky, rum, brandy, or whatever you like best. Add sugar to taste if you have a sweet tooth. Take the drink to bed but don't drink it until you are tucked in. As soon as you have drunk the last drop turn out the light and go to sleep. Do not add your tot to the milk until *after* it is boiled— if the liquor is added too soon the cure can't work.

TONIGHT'S TRIVIA

- Turtles have no teeth.
- Middle names were once illegal in England.
- Alaska has a longer coastline than that of all the lower forty-eight states combined.
- Back pain is the major cause of physical discomfort among Americans.

March 22

TONIGHT'S CURE

Orchestrated. Imagine you are a musician playing in the orchestra at Carnegie Hall in New York City. Choose one of your favorite pieces of music and hum it quietly to yourself. Begin by playing the piano part and move on to the violin, playing each instrument slowly as you go through the orchestra. Be sure to choose a soothing piece of music though—Peter Tchaikovsky's *1812 Overture* won't help you get to sleep!

TONIGHT'S TRIVIA

- An Indian poem called the *Mahabharata* contains nearly three million words.
- Homer was blind.

- The Romans worshipped a god called Robigus who protected their crops from mildew.
- Every year the collections in the New York Public Library increase by almost a million additions.

March 23

TONIGHT'S CURE

Fall asleep. Take more pillows than you normally use and prop them around you so you are in an upright, sitting position. Now stare straight in front of you until your eyes feel tired and start to close. Let your head drop forward if this feels more comfortable. Allow yourself to fall asleep in this position.

TONIGHT'S TRIVIA

- The compass was invented by Chou Kung, who had a swivel wrist.
- The game of bridge originated in Turkey.
- A Madame Schwartz from Berlin was able to understand words pronounced backward.
- The Belgian hare isn't a hare—it's a rabbit.

March 24

TONIGHT'S CURE

Nine hundred and ninety-nine. Lie back on the bed in a comfortable position. Start at nine hundred and ninety-nine and count backward until you reach one. If at any time you lose count, however, you have to go back to nine hundred and ninety-nine and start all over again.

TONIGHT'S TRIVIA

- In one year fifteen hundred Kenyans were killed by a pride of twenty-two lions.
- During the French Revolution pregnant shoplifters were given special consideration.
- An emu can run up to thirty miles per hour.
- There were more colonists for the British during the American revolution than for the Continental Army.

March 25

TONIGHT'S CURE

Stepping it up. If you live in a house with stairs walk up and down the stairs at least six times before retiring to bed. Once you're in bed imagine a very long spiral staircase and visualize yourself climbing up the steps. Keep going up and up and up until you feel exhausted. Then experience the pleasure of running down and down and down the steps and into a deep sleep.

TONIGHT'S TRIVIA

- A penguin swims using its wings as rudders.
- Mustard gas is not a gas but a liquid.
- In A.D. 401 the Black Sea was completely frozen over.
- During World War I patriotic Americans renamed sauerkraut "liberty cabbage."

March 26

TONIGHT'S CURE

Fresh air. Before getting into bed stand by an open window. Breathe in very deeply filling your lungs with fresh air. Hold your breath for ten seconds and then release it completely. Breathe in again very slowly, filling your lungs with as much air as they can take, and this time hold your breath for five seconds and exhale. Repeat this three times. Finally, breathe in and out very quickly ten times and get straight into bed.

TONIGHT'S TRIVIA

- It is only a century since corpses used to be stored in the cellars of public houses before burial.
- The jaguar catches fish with its paws.
- Butterflies taste with their feet.
- You can tell a fish's age by counting the rings on its scales.

March 27

TONIGHT'S CURE

Midnight mass. Imagine you are in church. Try to sense the peace and tranquility of the building and the atmosphere inside. Picture the beauty of the stained-glass windows. Try to visualize the statues and decoration. Listen to the choir singing one of your favorite hymns. Join in with them, humming the hymn softly to yourself.

TONIGHT'S TRIVIA

• Soldiers in ancient Greece used to go into battle naked from the waist down.
• An American heiress once left her fortune to provide clothes for snowmen.
• In Melbourne, Australia, chickens were used to control the traffic in 1975.
• On March 27, 1966, an earthquake registering 8.9 on the Richter Scale struck Alaska. In Anchorage the streets "rippled like waves." An entire village on Kodiak Island disappeared and one fishing boat was carried to a schoolyard five blocks inland. While all this happened Alaska's earthquake experts were down in Washington State at a conference—on earthquakes!

March 28

TONIGHT'S CURE

Conversation piece. Imagine having a conversation with a stranger who is visiting your city. Tell him or her a little about yourself, your lifestyle, your family, your job, and where you live. Explain the district and how to get to a certain place that he is seeking. Gradually let the stranger take over more and more of the conversation until you are listening entirely to what he or she has to say.

TONIGHT'S TRIVIA

• There is a breed of cow called Why.
• In Africa there is a snuffbox tree, the wood of which is used to make snuffboxes.
• In eighteenth century France coal miners were often women and children.
• During the American Revolution soldiers increased their height by wearing hats that were eighteen inches high.

March 29

TONIGHT'S CURE

Insomniac's cocktail. During the evening, not too soon before going to bed, make yourself an insomniac's cocktail. You will need one-third Campari, one-third sweet vermouth, and one-third gin. Mix this together with a little bit of ice and a slice of lemon to taste.

TONIGHT'S TRIVIA

- Clouds are higher at night than during the day.
- The oldest farm in Australia was built in 1794.
- Thomas Jefferson once had a life-mask made but the plaster set too soon and had to be chiseled from his face.
- A sixteenth century calendar has been discovered carved on the shoulder blade of an ox.

March 30

TONIGHT'S CURE

Farmer Brown. Farmer Brown has the unenviable task of taking across a river a fox, a goose, and a sack of corn. Unfortunately his boat will only hold him and one of the three. If left on their own either the fox will eat the goose or the goose will eat the corn. Before you attempt to fall asleep work out how you think Farmer Brown got all of them safely across. *

TONIGHT'S TRIVIA

- The first elevator was installed in a department store in 1857.
- An owl can eat ten mice in one meal.
- In Mali, Africa, there is a natural rock formation that looks like fingers pointing to heaven.
- On March 30, 1857, U. S. Secretary of State William H. Seward concluded one of the most crucial deals in U. S. history. He bought 586,400 square miles of land from Tsar Alexander II of Russia. The land was named Alaska and the cost worked out to less than two cents per acre.

*Farmer Brown takes the goose across, returns and takes the fox over, bringing the goose back with him. He then takes the corn across, returning to fetch the goose.

March 31

TONIGHT'S CURE

Jet setting. Imagine that you are in a jet flying off on an exotic vacation to the Caribbean with the love of your life. Feel the take-off whisking you up, up, and away and off into the wide blue yonder. Feel the release of tension as you undo your seat belt. Leave your worries behind and float off to the deep blue skies and the sun. Order a bottle of Dom Perignon champagne, relax in your seat, and imagine the tropical sunshine awaiting you at your destination.

TONIGHT'S TRIVIA

- $33 \times 3367 = 111{,}111$
  $66 \times 3367 = 222{,}222$
  $99 \times 3367 = 333{,}333$
  $132 \times 3367 = 444{,}444$ and so on until you reach
  $297 \times 3367 = 999{,}999$.
- In New Zealand a cow was once sentenced to two days imprisonment for eating the lawn outside a courthouse.
- Butterflies were originally called flutterbys.
- Whitcomb L. Judson of Chicago heralded reassurance for millions of men around the world on March 31, 1896. He patented the first zipper.

April 1

TONIGHT'S CURE

Telephone numbers. Take a sheet of paper. At the top write down your own telephone number. Then write down your office number and your mother's or close relative's number. Write down the number of the rest of your relatives followed by the numbers of your friends, and finally the numbers of your enemies. If it gives you satisfaction call one of your enemies and see if they are asleep! Write down as many telephone numbers as you can. The mental exercise will soon tire your brain sufficiently. But if it doesn't try to remember as many area codes as you can and list these in alphabetical order.

TONIGHT'S TRIVIA

- The first day of April is called "April Fool's Day" in England, "Doll Day" in Japan, "Boob Day" in Spain, and "Fish Day" in France.
- There are twelve metals heavier than lead: Gold, iridium, mercury, osmium, palladium, platinum, rhodium, rubidium, ruthenium, thalium, tungsten, and uranium.
- A French composer named Darius once composed an opera lasting seven and one-half minutes.
- In April 1749, Benjamin Franklin gave an electric picnic where the food was killed and cooked by electricity.

April 2

TONIGHT'S CURE

Objective thinking. If you have anything on your mind that is preventing you from sleeping, step back and look at the problem objectively to see if it really warrants so much worrying. During the day we're usually too preoccupied to take a rational look at our worries, but at night we can lie in the dark and analyze exactly why we're so high strung. If it helps, try to imagine you're hearing about this worry from someone else. Advise them how to solve the problem by putting their anxieties into perspective. Show how they've let things get out of proportion. Then switch back to being yourself and fall asleep.

TONIGHT'S TRIVIA

• In 1917 an Austrian woman, Mathilde Kovacs, revenged herself on her relatives who had been discourteous to her cats by setting fire to her entire fortune just before her death.
• Skin grafts can only be taken from another area of your body or an identical twin.
• Our body moves by using over six hundred muscles.
• A normal human brain weighs three pounds.

April 3

TONIGHT'S CURE

Lemon cure. Hot lemon juice is one of the most soothing nightcaps. All you have to do is cut a couple of slices from a lemon and then squeeze the rest of the juice into a cup or heat-proof glass. Pour in boiling water and add a little sugar if you can't take the straight lemon juice. Take the drink to bed with you and sip it very slowly to reap the full benefit.

TONIGHT'S TRIVIA

• Babies can breathe and swallow at the same time. Adults cannot.
• It is impossible to sneeze and keep your eyes open at the same time.
• The population of the world increases by 1.5 million every week.
• Jesse James was shot dead on April 3, 1882, and forty-two years later to the day Marlon Brando was born.

April 4

TONIGHT'S CURE

Flower power. Imagine what it's like to be a honey bee. Imagine yourself landing on the petals of a large flower. Look at the beautiful colors of the petals. Smell the delicious fragrance. Crawl inside the bloom towards the delicious pollen. Remember that some flowers are going to be as high as a horse and eating the pollen is going to be a glorious feast.

TONIGHT'S TRIVIA

- Brown eyes have more pigment than blue eyes.
- The human mouth produces three pints of saliva a day.
- Two-thirds of the body's weight is water.
- If a hunk of supernova star no bigger than a baseball were brought to earth it would be heavier than the Empire State Building.

April 5

TONIGHT'S CURE

Herbal tea. For many centuries herbal teas have been successful remedies for insomnia—they are nature's tranquilizers and are not addictive. A cupful half an hour before you go to bed will calm you down and ensure restful sleep. Health stores will sell all the varieties you need such as chamomile, catnip, skullcap, and passion-flower teas.

TONIGHT'S TRIVIA

- Walking quickly uses eight times more calories than writing.
- America gave the world tomatoes, tobacco, and tapioca.
- Casanova used to eat oysters for breakfast, often as many as fifty.
- Wheeled transport is one thousand years older than the road.

April 6

TONIGHT'S CURE

Muscle awareness. Make yourself comfortable by lying completely flat. Cover your body with light covers so that you are warm but not hampered by anything too heavy. Take a few deep breaths. Now concentrate on the muscles in your feet. Wiggle them about, consciously tell them to relax, and let them go limp. Focus your attention on each part of your body separately and tell it to go to sleep. Work upwards towards your head until your whole body becomes completely relaxed.

TONIGHT'S TRIVIA

- Redheads have fewer hairs than blondes.
- Muhammad Ali is the only man to have twice regained the world heavyweight boxing title.
- Rattlesnakes are eaten in Florida as an hors d'oeuvre.
- In Iraq you cannot eat snakes on a Sunday.

April 7

TONIGHT'S CURE

Massage. As you lie on your bed get someone to massage away all the tension. You can massage each other if you wish so that you both sleep well. The masseur should take a bottle of baby oil or lotion, pour a little into the palm of one hand, and massage it onto your body with very firm circular movements. He or she should be paying particular attention to the muscles of the neck and shoulder, gradually working down the spine pummeling and rubbing, using more oil as necessary. There are many books available on special massage techniques but these are not essential. You will soon discover which strokes you find most soothing and your masseur will soon discover new movements. You'll find that massage can be very relaxing, not only for the person being massaged but for the masseur as well.

TONIGHT'S TRIVIA

- Apricot oil is not only used in food but also in cosmetics.
- Poodles do not molt.
- On Mars a man would weigh 38 percent of his body weight on earth.
- *Nebuchadnezzar* is Russian for no God and no czar.

April 8

TONIGHT'S CURE

Boring book. Find the most boring book you can, preferably a paperback with very small print. Prop yourself up in bed and try to read it, attempting to interest yourself in the subject matter.

Eventually your eyes will become tired and you will find that you are unable to concentrate. Turn out the light and go to sleep. (Books in foreign languages work well provided you can't understand the language.)

TONIGHT'S TRIVIA

• Dandelion leaves are delicious in salads.
• In Siberia people display their love by throwing slugs and lice at each other.
• Mayflies live only a few hours when hatched.
• Bungalows are named after the Hindu word *bangla* which means belonging to Bengal.

April 9

TONIGHT'S CURE

Sweetheart. Lie back on your bed. Take a couple of deep breaths. Gently sway from side to side in a rocking motion. Choose an image of a person of whom you are very fond, or a person who makes you happy. Picture that person laughing. Hug yourself very tightly as you rock and imagine that person in your arms. Squeeze them very tightly. Don't let other thoughts intrude, and if they do, quickly bring back the image of your sweetheart.

TONIGHT'S TRIVIA

• If a person in Australia could shout loudly enough to be heard in New York, it would take fourteen hours for the sound of their voice to arrive in New York.
• The elephant is the only animal with four knees.
• An English novelist, Anna Marie Porter (b.1781), published her first novel at the age of eleven.
• There were only fifty men in the American Air Force at the outbreak of World War I.

April 10

TONIGHT'S CURE

Neck comforter. You need a hot-water bottle for this cure, ideally one covered with fur or some other fabric that will allow you to use almost boiling water. Get into bed and lie on whichever side you normally sleep. Now place the bottle across your shoulders and the base of your neck and feel the heat penetrating your tired muscles, gradually releasing all your tension.

- In 1868 the first traffic lights in England exploded, killing a policeman.
- Cars were first started with ignition keys in 1949.
- Thirty thousand tons of cosmic dust are deposited on the earth each year.
- More Americans have been killed in automobile accidents than in all the wars ever fought by the United States.

April 11

TONIGHT'S CURE

Total body relaxation. Relax your body completely, starting with your feet, by saying to yourself: "My feet are relaxing, they are tired, they are feeling heavy, they are completely relaxed." Move on to your legs, calves, and thighs. Do this for each part of the body including the neck, tongue, lips, eyes, and forehead. At the finish say: "My whole body is completely at peace, I am relaxed, all the tension has gone, I am warm." Now count backward from ten, relaxing more with each passing number: "Ten, I am letting go more and more, nine, I am feeling really calm," and so on until you reach one. You'll find that your whole body will tingle because the mental suggestion will lead you into a state of complete relaxation.

TONIGHT'S TRIVIA

- Kubla Khan invented a gunpowder-filled hand-grenade in 1230.
- The Dingo is the only native Australian animal that eats meat.
- One prong of male reindeer antlers protects its eyes during a fight.
- The star of the 1933 film *King Kong* was a hand-puppet only six-inches high.

April 12

TONIGHT'S CURE

Decanter. If your body is tired but your mind is overactive, as can often be the case, imagine that your body is a decanter. Breathe in very slowly imagining you are a decanter filling with rich red wine. Keep breathing in until you are full and hold the air for as long as you can. Then breathe out very slowly imagining you are a decanter being emptied very carefully. Once you're empty start the cycle again and repeat it five times.

TONIGHT'S TRIVIA

- There are 120 different species of buttercup.
- Fried mice used to be given in Britain as a cure for smallpox.
- The first shots of the Civil War were fired on April 12, 1861. Exactly four years later to the day the Confederate President, Jefferson Davis, was informed that the South had surrendered.
- Woodrow Wilson was the only U.S. president to hold a Ph.D.

April 13

TONIGHT'S CURE

Skiing. Imagine you are skiing down a dazzling mountain slope with the sunshine glistening on the snow and the sound of your skies hissing and swishing beneath you. You are wrapped up warmly and you can feel the warmth of the sun on your face and the freshness of the air. Start at the top of the slope and relax as you ski down and down and down in long swooping curves toward the green forest at the foot of the mountain.

TONIGHT'S TRIVIA

- The constitution of South Carolina was drafted by an English philosopher—John Locke.
- Greek and Roman statues were frequently decorated with inlaid accessories and many were made with detachable heads.
- The United States makes and uses over half the tin cans in the world.
- The "big cheese" comes not from cheese, but from the Hindu *chiz,* "thing."

April 14

TONIGHT'S CURE

Threesome. If insecurity keeps you awake try going to bed with two extra pillows. Place one on either side of you so you have room to move comfortably in between but also have reassurance of support and protection in front and behind just as if there were two other people to shelter you. If it makes you feel even more secure, pull the pillows closer to you so you are sandwiched right in between. You can even hug them if that helps you fall asleep.

- Joan of Arc was nineteen when she was burned at the stake.
- Four babies are born every second.
- Newborn ducks do not know how to swim.
- William Shakespeare spelled his name eleven different ways.

April 15

TONIGHT'S CURE

Autobiography. Tonight begin writing your autobiography. Take a notebook and pen and start with your earliest recollections. Take your mind back to your early childhood, even babyhood if you can remember back that far. However fragmented the memories may be, jot them down. Continue on from childhood working through your schooldays until you feel sleepy. You never know, you may wish to continue nightly from now on until it is completed.

TONIGHT'S TRIVIA

- The Greek word for pearl gave the name to a new food— margarine.
- The Romans called a sandwich *offula*.
- The oldest example of writing is found on a limestone tablet dated 3500 B.C.
- Guinea pigs aren't pigs and don't come from Guinea. They are domestic rodents which originate in South America.

April 16

TONIGHT'S CURE

Multiplication. Did you doze off during math lessons in school? If you did here's the cure for you. Recite your multiplication tables. Start with 1×12, 2×12, until you reach 12×12. Then go on to 1×13, 2×13, until you reach 13×13. Continue until you reach 25×25.

TONIGHT'S TRIVIA

- The oldest recorded human name is N'armer.
- Making love uses half as many calories as skipping.
- A church in Lorentz Weiler, Luxembourg, is located inside a cave.
- The exclamation point comes from the Greek *Io*, which means I am surprised, and which we have turned into I or !.

April 17

TONIGHT'S CURE

Scotch slumber. Place a lighted candle at the foot of your bed. Pour four ounces of whisky into an eight-ounce glass and add three teaspoons of sugar. Fill up the glass with boiling water, get into bed, and turn out the light. Sip this mixture while concentrating on the candle. As soon as three candles appear, blow out the middle one and lie down ready for sleep.

TONIGHT'S TRIVIA

• Brazil has more forests than anywhere in the world yet imports more timber than it exports.
• The Chinese were using stirrups two thousand years ago.
• The only Christians to use the Star of David on gravestones are the Basques.
• The average annual family income in the United States during 1915 was $687.

April 18

TONIGHT'S CURE

White sheet. If the total-blackness cure couldn't help you try the opposite—the white-sheet cure. Close your eyes. Imagine a large white sheet is hanging on a line in front of you. Walk right up to the sheet until you see nothing but white. Let this envelop you completely. Blot all other thoughts from your mind and concentrate on the whiteness. Look closely at the sheet, examine its texture and weave, try to count the individual threads, and finally, concentrate on the fibres in each thread.

TONIGHT'S TRIVIA

• In 1831 Giovanni Rubini, the Italian operatic tenor, sang a very high note with such force that he dislocated his collarbone.
• In Sweden mushrooms are protected by law.
• Wolfgang Mozart was composing and playing music at the age of four.
• On April 18, 1775, Paul Revere made his epic ride from Charleston to Lexington. On the other side of the continent, 131 years later to the day, San Francisco was devastated by the 1906 earthquake and fire.

April 19

TONIGHT'S CURE

Sleep tapes. It is now possible to buy sleep-inducing tape recordings that include such sounds as a human heart beat (said to have the peaceful effect of being in the womb before birth). However, making your own sleep tapes, by simply recording the most boring and montonous sounds you can think of, and playing them to yourself as you lie in bed can achieve the same goal.

TONIGHT'S TRIVIA

• The first foam rubber was made by beating latex in an electric food mixer.

• The town of Rugby, North Dakota, is the precise geographical center of the North American continent.

• The battle of Lexington, fought on April 19, 1775, had one of the lowest casualty lists of all time. Only eight men were killed.

• Only two U.S. presidents were outlived by their fathers— Warren G. Harding and John F. Kennedy.

April 20

TONIGHT'S CURE

Ritual change. Nearly all of us have a nightly ritual before going to bed; we brush our teeth, put the cat out, watch the TV news, and have a goodnight kiss, all at the same time every night. In many ways it is good to get into a routine because it prepares your body for sleep. But if you are an insomniac, then it might be wise to change your ritual just a little. Try drinking something different, changing your bedtime, or if you wear pajamas, try not wearing any. Try to make changes in every aspect of your bedtime routine—any one of them may be keeping you awake.

TONIGHT'S TRIVIA

• No one has ever died from insomnia.

• The English playwright, William Shakespeare, never saw an actress in his entire life. In those days all the parts were played by men.

• Typewriters were first developed to help the blind.

• A fully-grown walrus yields seventy gallons of pure oil.

April 21

TONIGHT'S CURE

Vowel trouble. As you lie awake, think of as many words as you can that contain all the five vowels—*a,e,i,o, and u*—preferably, but not necessarily, in that order. To start you off, here are two: abstemious and facetious. How many more can you think of?

TONIGHT'S TRIVIA

• A ball of black widow spider's web the size of a pea would be thirty miles long if straightened out.
• In scientific laboratories the color for danger is bright yellow.
• Blaise Pascal, a French mathematician and philosopher, invented a calculating machine when he was nineteen.
• There is a set of traffic lights in Venice at the junction of the canals.

April 22

TONIGHT'S CURE

Shakespeare. The calming effect of poetry can often help you fall asleep. Take a copy of Shakespeare's sonnets and start reading them out loud. Here is one sonnet to begin with if you haven't a copy. Read it aloud at least several times before you start to analyze its meaning.

> *The little Love-god lying once asleep*
> *Laid by his side his heart-inflaming brand,*
> *Whilst many nymphs that vow'd chaste life to keep*
> *Came tripping by; but in her maiden hand*
> *The fairest votary took up that fire*
> *Which many legions of true hearts had warm'd;*
> *And so the general of hot desire*
> *Was sleeping by a virgin hand disarm'd.*
> *This brand she quenched in a cool well by,*
> *Which from Love's fire took heat perpetual,*
> *Growing a bath and healthful remedy*
> *For men diseased; but I, my mistress' thrall,*
> *   Came there for cure, and this by that I prove,*
> *   Love's fire heats water, water cools not love.*

TONIGHT'S TRIVIA

- King Edward VIII of England is the only British monarch to have written his autobiography.
- Carpet beetles have lived in a bottle for two years eating nothing but their own dead skins.
- The earth's rotation on its axis causes any given point on the equator to travel 46.4 miles a minute.
- Weather vanes face in the opposite direction than that from which the wind is blowing.

April 23

TONIGHT'S CURE

Carefree days. If today's worries are keeping you awake tonight cast your mind back to the carefree days of your youth. Think about the happy days you had in school when your only worries were if your best friend would be wearing identical clothes. Think of all the activities you were involved in when you grew older: baseball, dance classes, vacations, and summer camps. Remember how excited you got when each birthday came round. Try to remember how free of worry life was then—and yet you still had bad days. Are things really so different now?

TONIGHT'S TRIVIA

- The human brain is four-fifths water.
- Noah was an albino.
- The official name for Libya is *Splaj.*
- According to tradition William Shakespeare was born on April 23, 1566, and died on his birthday in 1616.

April 24

TONIGHT'S CURE

Chinese prescription. The ancient Chinese had a cure for most things and this is what they recommended for insomnia. Mix freshly grated orange peel, extract of chopped ginseng, and honey. Add boiling water and drink the brew when you're in bed. This cure for insomnia has certain healing powers too. Maybe it's worth trying if you're sick even when you can snatch a few hours of sleep.

TONIGHT'S TRIVIA

- Benjamin Franklin was the youngest son of a youngest son of a youngest son.

- A dog turns around before going to sleep so that he faces the direction of the wind and can sense danger.
- Tin was the first metal used by man.
- A battleship requires two miles in which to turn around.

April 25

TONIGHT'S CURE

Clerical cats. Since many priests keep cats here's a mental exercise that should tire out even the most active brain. Take each letter of the alphabet in turn and name a clergyman and his cat's outstanding characteristic. For instance, the archbishop has an acrobatic cat, the bishop's cat is a boring cat, the cardinal's cat is a comical cat, the dean's cat is a dangerous cat, the evangelist's cat is an elegant cat, and so on until you reach Z.

TONIGHT'S TRIVIA

- The division of the day and night into equal sections was implemented four thousand years ago.
- A moth has no mouth and no stomach.
- There is a village called Hell near Trondheim, Norway.
- Dr. Guillotine's invention of a humane executioner was given its first practical demonstration on April 25, 1792. The first victim of the guillotine was a convicted highwayman.

April 26

TONIGHT'S CURE

Fifty-two. Close your eyes and picture a large figure 52. Look at the five and say "two". Look at the two and say "five". Repeat this five times concentrating on the numbers as you speak. By the time you come to the sixth repetition you ought to be falling asleep.

TONIGHT'S TRIVIA

- In 1790 Issaac Hibbitts died. He had been a bachelor until the age of seventy. From then until his death at the age of a hundred he married seven times, outlived six wives, and fathered children with each.
- The ancient Greeks invented insecticides from toxic chemicals.
- At a British public auction in 1832, a man sold his wife and dog as one "lot" for £1.
- Abraham Lincoln's son, Robert Todd Lincoln, was present at the

assassinations of three presidents: those of his father, President James Garfield, and President William McKinley.

April 27

TONIGHT'S CURE

What time? Gordon and Paul both go for a swim but unfortunately forget to remove their wristwatches. As a result both watches are damaged. Gordon's starts to gain thirty seconds a day and Paul's stops altogether. If they both decide never to set or repair their watches again, which of the two will tell the exact time more often, and how much more often?*

TONIGHT'S TRIVIA

- This tombstone is found in a British churchyard:
  Here lies in silent clay
  Miss Arabella Young
  Who for the first time this day
  Began to hold her tongue.
- At twenty-five thousand feet a pilot can see for 194 miles.
- There is a river in Colombia flowing with water that is so acidic it tastes like vinegar. In fact no fish can inhabit the water because it is so sour.
- A five-cent bill was once legal currency in America.

*Solution: For Gordon's watch to show the correct time again it will take 2 × 60 × 12 half days, i.e. 720 days. During this time Paul's watch will have shown the correct time twice daily, which is 1,440 times, which is 1,500 times more often than Gordon's.

April 28

TONIGHT'S CURE

Movie fun. Think of every motion picture you have seen, not on TV but at the movies. Put them in chronological order starting with the very first one you ever saw; perhaps it was a Disney cartoon, as a child or perhaps it was a western. No matter what it was start from there and work right through to the most recent movie you have seen. When you put them all in chronological order, if you can that is, choose the picture you enjoyed most and try to visualize it scene by scene from beginning to end.

TONIGHT'S TRIVIA

• A submarine cannot remain still at one depth and has to keep rising and falling.
• In 1884 a patent was taken out on a musical cigar in Germany.
• In New Orleans no burials are allowed because the ground is so damp. Instead mausoleums are used to house the dead.
• The human eye can distinguish 2 million different colors and shades.

April 29

TONIGHT'S CURE

Constructive criticism. If the cause of your insomnia is one particular person, and invariably it is, how about letting them know just how you feel. Write a letter telling exactly what you think about them or the trouble they're causing you. Be as cutting and as rude as you like so you will get your worries off your chest. Seal the envelope and turn off your light. (When you wake up just toss the letter in the garbage and have a good day.)

TONIGHT'S TRIVIA

• In 1812 a British clergyman began reading six chapters of the Bible every hour for one thousand consecutive hours. At the end of thirteen days and nights he fell into a profound sleep from which he never awoke.
• The Aztec civilization functioned without the wheel.
• The first equal sign (=) was published in 1557.
• Roman senators wore purple stripes on their togas as a sign of rank.

April 30

TONIGHT'S CURE

Cooling off. Perhaps you're too hot in bed. Is that what's keeping you awake? If it is try lying on your back after you have been in bed a little while. Hold the top of your blanket or quilt gently with both hands, lift it up about a foot, and then let it drop. Repeat this ten times making sure you let go completely each time. Fresh, cool air will circulate round the bed and you'll find it much more comfortable.

TONIGHT'S TRIVIA

• Uranus takes eighty-four years to orbit the sun.

• During the sixteenth century anyone attempting to leave Japan was executed.

• The Queen of Madagascar, who died in 1874, was buried in a coffin made of thirty thousand silver coins riveted together.

• April 30 has marked three major events in American history. In 1789 George Washington was inaugurated as the first president of the United States. In 1803 the United States bought a vast area of land from France, stretching from the Mississippi to Canada, at a little under three cents an acre. And in 1812 Louisiana (part of the former French territory) achieved statehood.

May 1

TONIGHT'S CURE

Lettuce sleep. Lettuce is said to have sedative power and many believe that eating lettuce for supper will help you sleep. An old New England remedy is to drink lettuce tea. To brew this you take the outside leaves of a large lettuce and put them into half a pint of boiling salted water. You let this simmer for fifteen to twenty minutes, then strain off the liquid and drink it immediately before going to bed.

TONIGHT'S TRIVIA

• The nine-banded female armadillo always bears four young, either four male or four female, but never a mixture of both sexes.

• Seven-and-a-half million tons of water evaporate from the Dead Sea every day.

• The button was originally developed as a decoration.

• India ink comes from China.

May 2

TONIGHT'S CURE

Chocolate challenge. Imagine you have a bar of chocolate three-blocks wide by eight-blocks long. What is the minimum number of breaks you would need to make in order to separate each block, if you are not allowed to double up pieces?*

TONIGHT'S TRIVIA

• The Romans used weasels to catch mice.

- Babe Ruth didn't start his baseball career as a hitter. He began as a pitcher and only later switched to hitting.
- A waterfall near Honolulu falls upwards. This is caused by prevailing winds which catch the falling water and blow it back over the cliff.
- William Howard Taft is the only U.S. president who also held the post of chief justice.

*Solution: To produce twenty-four separate pieces you will require twenty-three breaks.

May 3

TONIGHT'S CURE

Clueless crosswords. Draw a large square with a grid of nine lines inside it so the square contains eighty-one smaller squares. Now write a nine-lettered word across the top and a nine-lettered word down the left hand side (note that they will both have to start with the same letter). Fill in the rest of the square with as many words as you can, putting in blank squares where necessary, so you end up with a finished crossword puzzle minus the clues. Then if you still do not feel sleepy give each of the words a clue.

TONIGHT'S TRIVIA

- In 1842 4.8 percent of babies who died before their first birthday did so from teething.
- At a Baby Show in Springfield, Ohio, a judge defined a baby as an "Alimentary canal with a loud noise at one end and no sense of responsibility at the other."
- The USSR is larger than the entire continent of South America.
- The sun weighs 330,000 times as much as the earth.

May 4

TONIGHT'S CURE

Hop pillow. For hundreds of years insomniacs have been finding merciful peace and sleep on hop pillows which are still in use today. You can buy them at health stores or you can make your own by collecting and drying hops and sewing them into a small pillowcase mixed with equal amounts of feathers or foam particles. Hops contain an alkaloid called "lupine" which acts as a sedative but has no harmful side effects.

TONIGHT'S TRIVIA

• Thales Kastor, of Illinois, has written over five thousand letters to editors of newspapers and magazines.
• In England, during the nineteenth century, the fashion was for women to have pink cheeks, red lips, and perfect eyebrows tattooed on to their faces.
• Children in Siberia travel to school on dog-pulled skis.
• Until 1796 what is today the state of Tennessee was called Franklin.

May 5

TONIGHT'S CURE

Soapbox. Have you ever attended a political meeting, a party convention, or listened to political debates? Have you ever tried to speak publicly yourself on any political issues? If you haven't, here's your chance. As you lie awake in the dark choose a subject that you'd like to air your views on and start to compose your speech. Try to make what you say original and try to avoid the usual political clichés. It's not easy to come up with a good speech, in fact you're likely to fall asleep before you do.

TONIGHT'S TRIVIA

• The Angel Falls in Venezuela are over half a mile high.
• Forks only came into general use during the last century.
• The first Christmas tree was erected in Strasbourg in 1605.
• Blindworms aren't blind and aren't worms—they're legless lizards that can see.

May 6

TONIGHT'S CURE

Teetotaler's nightcap. What use is a nightcap if you don't drink? None at all—unless it's nonalcoholic, which is just what this one is. Here's a delicious teetotal nightcap to soothe you into oblivion.

Take the juice of one lemon and one orange (or grapefruit). Mix these together with two tablespoons of honey. Add boiling water and sip slowly just before going to bed.

TONIGHT'S TRIVIA

- A fish's heart has two chambers.
- In proportion to its size the feather is the strongest natural structure.
- Medieval Japanese women used to stain their teeth black to improve their beauty.
- From side to side, the Statue of Liberty's mouth measures three feet.

May 7

. . . .

TONIGHT'S CURE

Alcoholic beverage. Hop pillows featured earlier, but if you're the type who prefers liquid hops to dry hops, and hops inside to hops outside, have a glass of beer before you turn in. Strong beers, such as Guinness, are the most effective, but any ale will do. On the other hand you can steep a handful of hops in boiling water for fifteen to twenty minutes before straining them and drinking the juice.

TONIGHT'S TRIVIA

- The English author, Jonathan Swift, famous for his book *Gulliver's Travels* once refused to speak to anyone for a whole year.
- For the Indian Pachsi tribe divorce is quite simple—the husband breaks a straw and the marriage is dissolved.
- The amoeba eats by wrapping its body around the food.
- Cabinetmakers use sharkskin as sandpaper.

May 8

. . . .

TONIGHT'S CURE

Dog dreams. If you have a dog, watch how he settles down. Firstly, when it comes to sleeping, a dog puts all its worries to one side. If you don't own a dog watch a friend's dog or dogs you see in parks or yards. A lot can be learned from them—you'll rarely see insomniac canines.

Secondly, before going to sleep dogs turn around several times. They scrunch up their bedding to make it soft and push their noses and ears right into it before falling asleep. So when you get into bed wriggle around into a comfortable position, plump up the pillows so they are really soft, and bury your head in the pillows.

But most important of all, put those worries out of your mind until morning.

TONIGHT'S TRIVIA

- In North America it was once believed that minced beaver testicles cured a toothache.
- The earth rotates around the sun at a speed of 66,600 miles per hour.
- The first man executed in an electric chair took eight minutes to die.
- There is more copper in the brain and liver of a baby than an adult.

May 9

TONIGHT'S CURE

The Lord's Prayer. If you're not in the habit of reciting the Lord's Prayer at night, try it this evening. Say the prayer to yourself once. Then go through it from the beginning counting how many times you come across the letter *A*, the letter *B, C, D*, and so on, until you reach *Z*—if you make it that far.

TONIGHT'S TRIVIA

- The Chinese character for good depicts a mother and child side by side.
- There are over 80 million people in the world with the surname Chang.
- There are two thousand species of parsley.
- *Jesus* is Greek for the Hebrew *Joshua*, a name meaning Savior.

May 10

TONIGHT'S CURE

Vermont farmers' remedy. Farmers in Vermont have their own special cure for insomnia. They mix apple-cider vinegar with pure honey, take two teaspoons before going to bed, and repeat this dose for every half hour they are awake until they fall asleep.

TONIGHT'S TRIVIA

- Temperatures have been recorded in Montana that were ten degrees lower than those recorded at the North Pole.
- The last European witch was burned in 1782, in Switzerland.

- During the Indian Mutiny the British wrote secret messages in milk and lemon juice.
- Atilla the Hun was a dwarf.

May 11

TONIGHT'S CURE

Beautiful bloomers. Do flowers remind you of warm summer days, of balmy breezes that lull you to sleep on hot afternoons? If they do try working your way through the alphabet listing flowers alphabetically starting with *A* for anemone, *B* for bluebell, *C* for carnation, *D* for daffodil, and so on. Then when you reach *Z* say your list in reverse order, making sure you remember each flower.

TONIGHT'S TRIVIA

- The only state in the United States whose name has one syllable is Maine.
- The albatross is never seen within sight of the mainland.
- Gioacchino Rossini wrote thirty-seven operas in the first thirty-eight years of his life and then wrote nothing during his remaining thirty-nine years.
- The women of the Toda tribe of southern India get only two garments during their entire lifetime.

May 12

TONIGHT'S CURE

Reverse counting. Start with five hundred and count back to one in threes, so you count 497, 494, 491, 488, 485, 482, 479, 476, 473, and so on until you reach one. It takes some thinking and most people rarely reach half way before they are asleep.

TONIGHT'S TRIVIA

- The only U.S. president to marry while living in the White House was Grover Cleveland.
- At Anthill, near Lagos, Nigeria, there is a rock shaped like a church.
- Luella Geer of Ravenna, Ohio, was fitted with false teeth in 1895 and was still wearing the same plate, without any alteration, eighty years later.
- Dwight Eisenhower's parents were pacifists.

May 13

TONIGHT'S CURE

Valerian root. Valerian root is easily obtainable from any drugstore. Just add four ounces to two pints of cold water and soak it for twelve hours; when it's ready, bring to the boil, add the liquid to your bath water before going to bed, and have a long, soothing soak in the tub. Alternatively you can put the root in a cheesecloth bag and suspend it under the hot tap as you run your bath. Either way Valerian root will help ease away the day's aches and pains.

TONIGHT'S TRIVIA

• George III of England bought sixty-seven thousand books during his lifetime.
• A mayfly in Polish is *chrzaszcz*.
• The Lhopa tribe in Tibet used to celebrate a marriage by eating the bride's mother at the wedding feast.
• For a man to fly like a bird he would need a breastbone seventy-nine inches long.

May 14

TONIGHT'S CURE

Love making. Reaching an orgasm is said to be the most natural and powerful sedative in the world, if not one of the greatest cures for insomnia. There are hundreds of sex guides on the market if you feel the need for a little encouragement; in fact one can attempt a different position for every night of the year! Mae West once boasted that she made love to a man named Ted for fifteen hours, which would soon solve anybody's insomnia problem.

TONIGHT'S TRIVIA

• On May 14, 1939 Lina Medina gave birth to a healthy, bouncing baby in Lima, Peru. The mother was five years and eight months old at the time.
• Cocoa is thought to be an aphrodisiac.
• Catherine the Great advocated sex six times a day as a cure for insomnia, and Brigitte Bardot once modestly asserted that she "must have a man every night." Cleopatra is said to have made love to a hundred men in one night.
• Wyoming was the first state to grant voters' rights to women.

May 15

TONIGHT'S CURE

Log cabin. Tonight you can relive the pioneering adventures of the olden days. Imagine you are in a log cabin in a wild, remote area of the frontier lands. Outside there are wolves howling and stalking their prey. The snow is lashing the shutters and falling in deep drifts. But inside the cabin you are sitting in front of a roaring log fire wrapped in the arms of the one you love. Nothing can harm you. All is warmth and peace, you are protected and safe. Close your eyes and try to hear the crackle of the logs and feel the warmth of their blaze on your face.

TONIGHT'S TRIVIA

• An American colonel, Russell Farnham, walked from St. Louis to Leningrad in less than a year.
• The altitude limit for birds is roughly the same height as the summit of Mount Everest (29,141 feet above sea level).
• If you travel due north from the mouth of the Amazon River the first land you reach will be Greenland.
• Two U.S. firsts happened today. In 1602 the first white man stepped ashore in New England, and in 1918 the United States inaugurated the world's first regular air mail service.

May 16

TONIGHT'S CURE

Up and down. Read these two problems, then put out the light and work out the solutions:

1. If you place a word in front of up and in front of down you get two expressions which have exactly the same meaning. What is the word?*

2. What is it that the man who makes it does not need, the man who buys it does not use, and the man who uses it does so without realizing it?*

TONIGHT'S TRIVIA

• Eighty percent of the rose species on earth come from Asia.
• At the present rate of erosion scientists estimate that the Niagara Falls will disappear in twenty-five thousand years.

- Table tennis was originally called gossamer.
- The oldest surviving contraceptive sheaths were made of sheep gut.

May 17

. . . .

TONIGHT'S CURE

Ambition. Let your wildest dreams come true tonight. Indulge your most closely guarded secrets. Close your eyes and realize one of your greatest ambitions. Perhaps you've always wanted to pilot the Concorde; if so, imagine yourself at the controls soaring fifty thousand feet through the air at Mach 2. Maybe you see yourself as a ballet dancer, a cabaret star, appearing in Las Vegas, or a daredevil freefall parachutist. Imagine what it would be like to actually achieve your ambition. Sense the thrill of doing the impossible, and imagine the excitement and adulation of your admirers as you complete your ambition to perfection. Bask in the thrill and the glory and fall peacefully asleep.

TONIGHT'S TRIVIA

- Ducks only lay eggs in the morning.
- In *One Hundred Days of Sodom* the Marquis De Sade catalogued six hundred different ways of making love.
- Rainbows only occur when the sun is at an angle of less than forty degrees above the horizon.
- A cat can draw its claws back in sheaths on its paws.

May 18

. . . .

TONIGHT'S CURE

Slippery Elm Food. Mix three heaping teaspoons of Slippery Elm Food with sugar and water to make a paste, then gradually stir in half a pint of cold milk. Place the mixture in a saucepan and allow it to boil, stirring the liquid the whole time. (You will need to bring it to the boil at least three times as the Slippery Elm will swell.) Drink the mixture every night for ten nights just before you go to bed. It is an acquired taste, but after a few nights you will find that you really enjoy Slippery Elm and that it helps you sleep.

TONIGHT'S TRIVIA

• When Mohammed Ali ruled Egypt his army was made up of one-eyed soldiers.

• Queen Elizabeth I of England had over two thousand gowns.

• Mercury is the only liquid element. Its specific gravity is greater than iron, meaning that a piece of iron will float on mercury.

• Riding a piebald horse was once considered a cure for whooping cough.

May 19

TONIGHT'S CURE

Bed socks. One of the most common, but least appreciated, causes of insomnia is cold feet. Cold feet cause bad circulation which in turn keeps you awake. Fortunately the remedy is simple—good old-fashioned bed socks. These keep your feet warm and cozy thereby improving your circulation. Of course if you don't have any bed socks, why not tackle tonight's insomnia by starting to knit yourself a pair?

TONIGHT'S TRIVIA

• Eighteenth century criminals were used as guinea pigs for smallpox vaccinations.

• In Borneo natives use salad bowls shaped like dogs, believing it will prevent indigestion.

• A frog has no neck so it cannot turn its head.

• Abraham Lincoln, the tallest U.S. president (six feet four inches tall), was exactly a foot taller than James Madison, the shortest U.S. president.

May 20

TONIGHT'S CURE

Nostril inhaling. It's best to sit up in bed to do this exercise, but if you happen to wake up in the night you can do it lying down. Place your right thumb over your right nostril closing it up completely so you breathe only through your left. Breathe in and out very slowly. holding the breath for three to five seconds when you breathe in. When you want to exhale, breathe out through your right nostril, lifting your thumb, at the same time blocking your left nostril by squeezing slightly with your middle ring finger. Now inhale through the right nostril, hold your breath and breathe out through the left. Then breathe in through the left, hold your breath and breathe out through the right again. Continue in this manner until you feel sleepy.

TONIGHT'S TRIVIA

• Cacti in the Sahara can survive over three years without water.
• Alexandre Gustave Eiffel, who engineered the Eiffel Tower, also engineered the steel interior skeleton of the Statue of Liberty.
• On May 20, 1927, Charles Lindbergh set out from Garden City, New York on the first solo nonstop transatlantic flight. He had to look through a periscope for the whole flight, because the plane's huge fuel tanks obscured his view. Sighting a fishing boat for the first time, Lindbergh was so excited that he cut his engine and shouted to the crew, "Which way is Ireland?" They were so amazed they couldn't answer.
• In 1936 Jesse Owens beat a horse in a hundred yard dash.

May 21

TONIGHT'S CURE

Unicorns. Lie on your back and let your mind wander. You can think of absolutely anything—*except unicorns*. Sounds easy, right? But you will find that the sheer effort of trying not think of unicorns will send you off to sleep before you even realize.

TONIGHT'S TRIVIA

• Milk is heavier than cream.
• Toulouse Lautrec had an excessively large penis.
• Audiences first began to pay for concert seats in 1672.
• Any fine dust, including flour, is liable to explode in a confined space because of a combination of oxygen and heat.

May 22

TONIGHT'S CURE

Sleep breathing. Try and copy the breathing pattern that occurs when you are in a deep sleep. This breathing tends to come from the back of the throat and usually induces people to snore if they lie on their backs. Try to imitate this breathing, and even snore if you have to—just concentrate on letting yourself relax to the rhythm of your breath.

- Fires in redwood forests actually occur inside the trees—the bark of the redwood tree is fireproof.
- The ring-tailed lemur makes the same sound as a cat.
- Rhubarb is a vegetable.
- Alexandre Bizet, composer of the opera *Carmen*, was so worn out by the rehearsals that he died three months later aged just thirty-six.

May 23

TONIGHT'S CURE

Self-hypnosis. Now is your chance to put into practice all those hypnotic tricks that have mesmerized you on TV or in the theater. Lie in a comfortable sleeping position and repeat slowly and clearly to yourself: "I am going to sleep, I am feeling tired, I am getting heavier and heavier, falling deeper and deeper. I am beginning to sleep. My eyes are really heavy. My legs are heavy. My body is heavy. I am getting sleepier and sleepier and sleepier" until you drift off to sleep.

TONIGHT'S TRIVIA

- The backbone of a camel is perfectly straight.
- Ancient Egyptian princesses wore corsets.
- Cucumbers, pumpkins, and tomatoes are fruits.
- Only one-quarter of a nickel is made of nickel, the rest is copper.

May 24

TONIGHT'S CURE

Eye focus. In this cure lie back and close your eyes. Now, keeping them closed, focus them as you would if you were looking towards the tip of your nose. Concentrate on holding this position even though your eyes are shut. Imagine that you are looking at your nose and try to picture what it looks like. Now, still keeping your eyes closed, focus them on your hairline, and try to visualize this as you did your nose. Now alternate between these two focal points, concentrating on each in turn until you feel yourself growing tired.

TONIGHT'S TRIVIA

- Glues, plastics, paints, and explosives can all be made from soybeans.
- Marie de Medici, Queen of France, owned a dress which at present day prices would cost $12 million. She wore it only once.
- Peter the Great could break silver coins with his fingers.
- George Washington was a champion wrestler and long jumper.

May 25

TONIGHT'S CURE

Muscle clenching. Lie back on your bed, lightly covered with the blankets, clench both your fists, hold them taut for twenty seconds, and then relax them. Now lift your head up off the pillow and hold it up for twenty seconds before relaxing. Now lift your feet three inches in the air, hold them up for twenty seconds, and then relax them. When you've finished repeat the cycle five to ten times and at the end your muscles will be loose and relaxed.

TONIGHT'S TRIVIA

- Louis XIV and Napoleon Bonaparte were born with teeth.
- King Solomon had seven hundred wives.
- The most frequently used word in our language is *the*.
- On May 25, 1935, U.S athlete Jesse Owens broke the world records for 100 yards, 220 yards, 220-yard low hurdles and the long jump, all in the space of forty-five minutes.

May 26

TONIGHT'S CURE

Perfume. Place a delicious, relaxing fragrance beside your bed. Perhaps this would be a scented candle which you can burn, some mild incense, a favorite perfume, or even a vase of your favorite flowers (there is no truth in the belief that flowers are harmful in a bedroom at night). Close your eyes and concentrate on the smell. Let your mind wander through the many beautiful thoughts and memories that you associate with the smell and savor the happy recollections as each one comes before your eyes.

TONIGHT'S TRIVIA

• Frederick the Great, of Prussia, used to drink coffee made with champagne.
• Queen Victoria was a carrier of hemophilia.
• Medical students increase their vocabulary by ten thousand words during their training.
• The legendary Italian film star Maciste could open a can of sardines by squeezing it with his fingers.

May 27

TONIGHT'S CURE

Richard Nixon's remedy. This remedy has been used by many U.S. presidents—including Gerald Ford, Jimmy Carter, and Ronald Reagan—when they've been unable to sleep. They all tried to remember the names and dates of their predecessors in chronological order, starting with George Washington 1789-97, John Adams 1797-1801, Thomas Jefferson 1801-09, James Madison 1809-17, James Monroe 1817-25, John Quincy Adams 1825-29, until the present day. So all you have to do is to imagine that you are the president of the United States and try to recount the names and dates of your predecessors.

TONIGHT'S TRIVIA

• On New Year's Day, 1907, President Theodore Roosevelt shook hands with 513 people.
• The bathtub used in the White House by President William Howard Taft was so big that four workmen could sit in it quite comfortably.
• James Knox Polk, the eleventh U.S. president, fulfilled all his election promises, but was the first president to refuse to stand for reelection.
• At age seventy-eight Andrew Jackson became the first president to have his photograph taken.

May 28

TONIGHT'S CURE

Sauna. If you've ever been in a sauna then you know how good you feel when you come out, with all your tensions soothed away; you feel clean and calm. So before you go to bed tonight give yourself a facial sauna. Fill a large bowl with boiling water and add a few drops of angelica or chamomile. Now place a large towel over the bowl, sit in front of it, and lift the towel over your head so your face is directly above the water and the steam is circulating round your eyes, nose, and mouth. You'll need to lift the towel occasionally to breathe, but try to bear it for as long as you can. After ten minutes come out of the minisauna. Splash your face with cold water and gently pat it dry before you go to bed.

TONIGHT'S TRIVIA

• The uniform and equipment worn and carried by soldiers in World War I was actually heavier than a suit of armour worn by knights of old.

•
$$
\begin{array}{r}
1\ 2\ 3\ 4\ 5\ 6\ 7\ 8\ 9 \\
9\ 8\ 7\ 6\ 5\ 4\ 3\ 2\ 1 \\
1\ 2\ 3\ 4\ 5\ 6\ 7\ 8\ 9 \\
9\ 8\ 7\ 6\ 5\ 4\ 3\ 2\ 1 \\
+\ 2 \\
\hline
2\ 2\ 2\ 2\ 2\ 2\ 2\ 2\ 2\ 2
\end{array}
$$

• The duckbilled platypus is the only animal with poisonous glands.

• The United States was still the world's number-one oil producer as recently as the early 1960s.

May 29

TONIGHT'S CURE

Limericks. As you lie awake, make up a limerick about each member of your family. If you're still awake, after that move on to your friends, boss, and co-workers. Here's one to get you going:

There was once a man known as Keith,
Who sat on his set of false teeth.
Said he, with a start,
"Oh Lor! Bless my heart!
I have bitten myself underneath!"

TONIGHT'S TRIVIA

• In an English churchyard reads the following tombstone:
Here lie the remains of Thomas Nicolls,
Who died in Philadelphia, March 1578.
Had he lived, he would have been buried here.

• Kangaroos are only one inch high at birth.

- The longest words in the Bible are *commandments* and *testimonies*.
- In New Zealand there are twenty sheep for every human inhabitant.

May 30

TONIGHT'S CURE

Dancing. One of the best ways to relieve tension and burn up excess energy is dancing. Get yourself ready for bed and then switch on the radio or a cassette player and start dancing around the bedroom. It doesn't matter if you do a fox-trot, a samba, or the latest disco dance, but obviously the more energetic dances are best. Get your partner to join in as well and make it a really fun way to tire yourselves out before you fall into bed and pass out.

TONIGHT'S TRIVIA

- You can make an egg stand on one end by shaking it violently so the broken yolk settles at the bottom. This trick was even performed by Christopher Columbus in front of the entire Spanish court.
- There are 35,740,800 deaths annually around the world.
- The shape of the letter *O* has remained unchanged for three thousand years.
- The scientific name for a werewolf is lycanthrope.

May 31

TONIGHT'S CURE

Pillow change. Whatever your pillows are made of, change them tonight. If they are feather, change to foam. If you use a solid foam pillow then change to one filled with foam pieces, and so on. Pillows also come in many different shapes and one that's claimed to be very good for inducing sleep is a cigar-shaped pillow. Try changing the number of pillows you have too. Lastly change your pillow cases, change cotton for linen ones and vice versa. You'll be amazed at the difference a few simple changes like these can make.

TONIGHT'S TRIVIA

- Elephants cannot jump.

- Japan's sacred mountain, Fujiyama, actually bends in the wind owing to the lightness of its structure.
- Johann Sebastian Bach wrote an opera about coffee.
- One house catches fire in the United States every forty-five seconds.

June 1

TONIGHT'S CURE

Beethoven. Music is a great soother as you've discovered already. But some music is especially effective. Take Beethoven's Piano Sonata No. 14 for example, the famous *Moonlight*. Try playing this softly by your bed while you're lying in the dark. The music was originally written to suggest Lake Lucerne by moonlight, so just let your imagination wander to some idyllic setting.

TONIGHT'S TRIVIA

- The great blue heron catches fish by spearing them with its beak.
- Japanese cherry blossoms come in fifty different varieties.
- A quarter has 119 grooves on its circumference—only one more groove than a dime.
- A natural rock formation on Phillip Island, Australia, looks like two elephants.

June 2

TONIGHT'S CURE

Coronation cure. On June 2, 1953, Queen Elizabeth II was crowned Queen of the United Kingdom, Australia, her other Realms and Territories, Head of the Commonwealth, and Defender of the Faith. Tonight, if you lie awake, try to remember all the monarchs of Great Britain from William the Conqueror to the present day. If you do not know them, then find a book and learn them tonight and see how many you remember the next time you're lying awake.

TONIGHT'S TRIVIA

- Queen Elizabeth I was the first monarch to install a WC in her home.
- King George V had the right to wear one hundred military and naval uniforms.
- Queen Elizabeth II is the great-granddaughter of Alfred the Great thirty-six times removed.

• The coronation ceremony for English monarcl
virtually unchanged since St. Dunstan crowned E
Whit Sunday in 973.

June 3

TONIGHT'S CURE

Night light. Some lights can be very comforting in a bedroom, particularly to those who had lights in their rooms as children. If you were one of those children try having a colored light beside your bed to help you fall asleep. You can put a nightlight in a colored glass so that it bathes the room in a warm glow. You'll know it's worked when you wake up for the first time and find the nightlight still burning. Just blow it out and go back to sleep. (If you want you can buy small electric lights with colored bulbs that have the same effect.)

TONIGHT'S TRIVIA

• In Albania a stamp was issued in honor of Ahmed Zogu I who achieved the dubious distinction of smoking 240 cigarettes a day.
• In Australia the stump-tailed lizard has a tail that looks like its head.
• Only 28 percent of solar eclipses are total eclipses of the sun.
• Adrienne Cuyot of Belgium was engaged 652 times and married 53 times over a period of less than twenty-five years.

June 4

TONIGHT'S CURE

Siesta. If not sleeping at night is your problem, how about taking a tip from the Latin countries and having a siesta in the afternoon? You might think that this will keep you from sleeping at night, but that's not the case. Sleeping eight hours at a stretch is only a social convenience, it's actually better for us to take our rest in two shorter periods. What's more, if you have a rest in the afternoon, you can go to bed much later and have a couple of extra hours in which to relax and unwind.

TONIGHT'S TRIVIA

• In early measurements a pace was a double step.
• In London, in 1907, an actress called Clare Bloodgood committed suicide because her co-star received better reviews.

...e days before bedsprings were invented, a rope was laced ...ss the bed frame and a small wrench was used to tighten up the ...ope when it sagged.

- Thomas Jefferson considered a staircase a waste of space, hence his Virginia home had only two very narrow staircases.

June 5

TONIGHT'S CURE

Clock change. One very effective way of altering your regular routine is to have a friend or someone in your family change the time on every clock in your house, including your watch. Then you have to follow this time and will probably find that your body will soon adjust to it and will only send you off to sleep when you're tired. Make sure, however, that the person who changes the clocks wakes you up at the correct time in the morning!

TONIGHT'S TRIVIA

- Polynesian divers in Tonga used to hold underwater walking races.
- Aristotle believed that honey fell with dew.
- Mrs. Euphemia Johnson was drinking her afternoon tea when she suddenly burst into flames. Her body burnt so quickly that her charred remains were found inside her unburned clothes.
- Mosquitoes can fly even when they are carrying a load of blood that is twice their own body weight.

June 6

TONIGHT'S CURE

Rooms. Take a tour of your house or apartment tonight, without leaving your bed. Test your memory to see how good your powers of observation are. Start by visualizing one room. Imagine walking through the door and what immediately faces you. Look at the wall covering, study it carefully, feel its texture. Look at the carpet, can you remember the exact pattern and coloring? Now look to your left and move systematically around the room trying to visualize each object and piece of furniture.

TONIGHT'S TRIVIA

- A camera marketed in France in 1882 was shaped like a gun.

- The male midwife toad carries the eggs on its back.
- In 1779 a fifty-five-dollar note was issued.
- In Bali the groom must help the bride cook the entire wedding feast.

June 7

TONIGHT'S CURE

Diaphragm breathing. Diaphragm breathing comes naturally to some people, but to others it can be quite hard. If you place the palms of your hands just below your ribs your palms should be covering your diaphragm. Hold them there so your fingertips are lightly touching your body and watch how they move when you breathe. As you inhale, if you are breathing from your diaphragm, your fingertips should be pulled slightly apart and forced together again as you exhale. Lie back and practice breathing from your diaphragm, feeling the regular rhythm with your fingers.

TONIGHT'S TRIVIA

- The longest word in the *Oxford English Dictionary* is *Floccinaucinihilipilification* which means the act of estimating that something is worthless.
- America is named after Amerigo Vespucci, the Italian explorer who, in 1499, was the first to discover the American mainland.
- There are seven hundred species of gourd.
- Julius Caesar was an epileptic.

June 8

TONIGHT'S CURE

Girls' names. You probably have favorite girls' names of your own, but can you think of one girl's name for every letter of the alphabet, starting with *A* for Arabella, *B* for Beatrice, *C* for Clarissa, *D* for Diedre, *E* for Ermintrude, through *Z* for Zena or Zelda? If you can do it with one name, try it with two, or even three.

TONIGHT'S TRIVIA

- The Chinese character for East is the combination of the symbols of sun behind tree.
- The sun burns 240 million tons of hydrogen dust every minute.

- Female ticks lay five thousand eggs at a time.
- Mark Twain made a fortune as a writer, but lost it as an inventor.

June 9

TONIGHT'S CURE

Forehead concentration. Take a piece of scotch tape or a small piece of self-adhesive paper. (It is possible to buy small adhesive colored circles which are best.) Stick the tape, or piece of paper, to your forehead, and then lie back on the bed and concentrate on this spot. First sense its presence. Then imagine that it is not there at all, and try to visualize your forehead minus the spot. Concentrate hard until you can no longer feel it sticking to your forehead. You should then be asleep.

TONIGHT'S TRIVIA

- The ancient Greeks had a system of issuing theater tickets so that seats could be reserved.
- A lead pencil will write an average of forty-five thousand words.
- At the age of twelve, Ellen Elizabeth Benson, of New York, had an IQ of 214.
- Celebrated artist John Kane started his career by decorating houses.

June 10

TONIGHT'S CURE

Vacation plans. Use tonight's sleepless hours to plan your vacation. Perhaps you've got a vacation coming up, in which case you can make real plans. But even if your vacation tonight is pure invention, it doesn't matter—it's the planning that counts. Plan the vacation of your dreams—a world cruise, a trip to the Orient, sailing down the timeless Nile past the tombs of Pharaohs long dead, or even a trip into space on board the shuttle. It doesn't matter where you travel or what you plan to do, just concentrate on all the details of the trip. What will you take? What will you wear? How will you travel? The list is almost endless, and you should be asleep before you reach the end.

TONIGHT'S TRIVIA

- The most beautiful white statues we have found from ancient times were originally covered with gold and precious stones.

- Money paid as a ransom to a kidnapper is tax deductible.
- In 1387 a gun was invented with 144 barrels—the early machine gun.
- Of the first twenty-three astronauts to fly on U.S. space missions all but two were either only children or first born sons.

June 11

TONIGHT'S CURE

Crossword. One of the simplest cures for insomnia is to take a newspaper or magazine to bed with you that contains a crossword puzzle. Start the puzzle and do not put out the light until you have completed, or at least attempted, every clue.

TONIGHT'S TRIVIA

- A World War II U.S. soldier, Alfred Blazis, could throw a grenade almost two-hundred eighty-five feet.
- In 1901 New York made it compulsory for all motor vehicles to be licensed—the first state to pass such a law.
- The British X certificate was introduced in 1951.
- The word *bully* has nothing to do with a bull, it comes from the Dutch term for lover, *boel.*

June 12

TONIGHT'S CURE

Boy's names. Just as you might have earlier tried to find one girl's name for every letter of the alphabet, now start with *A* for Alfred and work right through the alphabet finding a boy's name for every single letter. When you reach *Z* for Zachary, work backwards towards *A* with a completely different list of names.

TONIGHT'S TRIVIA

- Jack the Ripper was left-handed.
- In 1800 a portable shower for travelers was invented in France.
- On June 12, 1957, the twenty-five stone Olympic and professional weightlifting champion Paul Anderson of Toccoa, Georgia, lifted the equivalent weight of two large cars on his back, a total of 6,279 pounds.

• It took over four thousand years for the last ice sheet that covered the United States to melt. The ice was a mile deep.

June 13

TONIGHT'S CURE

Performances. Tonight's the night to cast your mind back and relive all the shows and concerts you've ever attended. Try to remember, in chronological order, everything you have seen performed live in a theater or concert hall—the plays, operas, ballets, concerts, and recitals—from your early teenage years through the present. What was the first play you ever saw? How did you feel when the houselights dimmed and the curtain rose? See if you can remember every occasion and the sensations you associate with those occasions.

TONIGHT'S TRIVIA

• A fly moves its wings at a rate of 330 beats a second.
• A dragonfly can see a gnat coming at a distance of eighteen feet.
• Male moths can detect a female moth six miles away by their smell.
• An American actor, Rondo Hatton, was so ugly that he played monsters in horror films without makeup.

June 14

TONIGHT'S CURE

House work. If you don't feel sleepy when bedtime comes around you could usefully start doing tomorrow's housework. Dusting, polishing, cleaning, and sweeping will all tire you and make you ready for bed, and there's the added bonus that they will save you a great deal of time the following day. Of course if you feel too tired to do housework then you will not be troubled by insomnia.

TONIGHT'S TRIVIA

• The earth is 5.517 times denser than water.
• Nero's wife Poppea wore face masks made from bread crumbs and asses' milk in bed each night.
• Combs were first used around 1000 B.C.
• In the early days of the California Gold Rush prospectors were paying as much as $7 for a glass of whisky in San Francisco.

June 15

TONIGHT'S CURE

Nocturne. The most soothing and soporific music ever written is a series of nocturnes by the great composer Frederic Chopin. A record or cassette of his nocturnes is a good investment for any insomniac, and played quietly each evening before going to bed should relieve any tension.

TONIGHT'S TRIVIA

• A single drop of water contains 100 billion atoms.
• In sixteenth and seventeenth century England ladies wore their wedding rings on their thumbs.
• The secretary bird can swallow a hen's egg whole without breaking the shell.
• In Perth, Australia, there are a group of natural rocks that look like tombstones.

June 16

TONIGHT'S CURE

Touring. If you're lying awake tonight here's an opportunity to tour every place you've ever visited, in alphabetical order. You can start by listing the countries you've visited, then the states, and gradually work down to counties and cities. (Make sure you maintain alphabetical order.)

TONIGHT'S TRIVIA

• In September, 1944, a Brooklyn lawyer left over $50,000 to his tiger cat.
• Painter James Mayo (1500-1555) had a beard so long that he could tread on it.
• Ninety members of Columbus's crew were convicts.
• Nitwits may be witless, but the word comes from the Dutch *niet wit,* "I don't know."

June 17

TONIGHT'S CURE

Young relations. Offer to have some young children stay with you, perhaps a new born baby, or two or three children who will be awake before seven A.M. and full of go all day. After only a few days you will experience absolutely no problems in falling asleep at night.

TONIGHT'S TRIVIA

• As recently as the eighteenth century, caterpillars were excommunicated from Pont-du-Chateau, France.
• The pens with which the Treaty of American Independence was signed in 1782 realized £500 at an auction sale in London in 1891.
• Kern, the architect of the famous St. Basil's church in Moscow, had his eyes put out by Ivan the Terrible in order to prevent him from building a similar church elsewhere.
• On June 17, 1872, Johann Strauss II conducted one of the most unusual concerts in American history. A choir of 20,000, an orchestra of 987 musicians, and 100 fellow conductors complete with binoculars were led through the evening's program by Strauss who conducted with an illuminated baton from the top of a lookout tower.

June 18

TONIGHT'S CURE

Here is the news. If you haven't read all your paper by the time you go to bed, take the paper with you. Begin with the front page and read every single word out loud until you've read every article. Then turn to page two and do the same. Work your way through the newspaper in this way until you feel really tired, only then turn out the light and try to fall asleep.

TONIGHT'S TRIVIA

• The chamois is able to stand on a circle measuring less than two inches in diameter.
• A hot-water pipe will freeze more readily than a cold-water pipe.
• Ninety-nine percent of the world's bromine comes from the sea.
• On June 18, 1880, red, white, and blue hailstones fell in Moscow.

June 19

TONIGHT'S CURE

Waterskiing. Even if you've never waterskied in your life, you can still imagine the sensation of being towed behind the boat across the surface of the clear, blue sea. You can imagine the warm sun on your body. You can imagine the tingling of the fine spray on your body and the warm wind rushing through your hair. Close your eyes and go waterskiing in your mind right now.

TONIGHT'S TRIVIA

• An armless golfer, Tom MacAuliffe from Buffalo, played eighteen holes in ninety-eight strokes. He gripped the club between his chin and his shoulder.

• An egg weights 40 percent more when freshly laid than just before it is hatched.

• One ounce of gold can be beaten by hand into gold leaf sufficient to cover an acre.

• Spades in a deck of cards have nothing to do with spades, the word comes from the Spanish *espada,* "sword."

June 20

TONIGHT'S CURE

Wash and brush up. Go to bed at your usual time tonight and try to get to sleep. If you can't, or if you wake up in the middle of the night, get up and go to the bathroom. Splash cold water all over your face and then pat it dry with a soft towel. Now sit in front of your mirror and brush your hair at least fifty times, brushing it all forward, then brushing it all back, before you go back to bed refreshed and ready for sleep.

TONIGHT'S TRIVIA

• The great pyramid of Cheops was the highest building in the world for four thousand years.

• The Empire State Building contains seven miles of life shafts.

• There are more than one billion galaxies in the whole universe.

• King John I of France reigned for four days.

June 21

TONIGHT'S CURE

Discordant sounds. If peaceful, soothing sounds can't help you get to sleep, try the exact opposite. Buy or make a tape recording of as many discordant sounds as you can—from bangs and crashes, to gunfire, wild animal cries, fireworks, and discordant music— sounds which will make it absolutely impossible to sleep. Play this tape for at least half an hour and then turn it off. Afterwards the peace and silence will be pure bliss and you'll fall asleep with no difficulty.

TONIGHT'S TRIVIA

- Flying neutrons from the blast of an atomic bomb reach a velocity of millions of miles an hour.
- In a millionth of a second 10,000,000,000,000,000,000,000,000,000 (10 octillion) explosive neutrons are released from one pound of uranium.
- In 1386 a judge in Falaise, France, condemned a sow to be mutilated and hanged for having killed a child. The sow was executed in the public square dressed in man's clothes.
- On the average a hundred people in the United States over the age of fourteen attempt suicide every day.

June 22

TONIGHT'S CURE

Spine massage. Massaging the spine can be very relaxing, but what do you do if you're alone? Here's the answer. Lie flat on your back on the floor. Lift your knees up toward your chest and clasp your arms around them. Then rock from side to side and in a circular motion and feel the base of your spine being massaged. It is a wonderfully soothing feeling.

TONIGHT'S TRIVIA

- Spiders spin their webs at night.
- In Madagascar spiders's web silk is woven into cloth.
- It is possible to pull a piece of wire through a block of ice with the block remaining in one piece.
- A hat worn by Napoleon brought almost two-thousand English pounds at an auction in London in 1891.

June 23

TONIGHT'S CURE

Speaking clock. If it's loneliness that keeps you awake during the night, telephone one of the recorded telephone message services. There are dozens to choose from; dial-a-disc, a recorded weather report, you can even dial you horoscope. If you want a conversation you could call a number in your area which will give you the time. You can say exactly what you want, and it won't hang up!

TONIGHT'S TRIVIA

- In 1683 the River Thames in London became completely frozen over and a Frost Fair was held on it.

- In 1697 it was recorded that a substance like butter fell from the air in the County of Limerick, Ireland.
- John Tyler, tenth U. S. president, entered the College of William and Mary at the age of twelve.
- Four future presidents attended the inauguration of Abraham Lincoln. They were Benjamin Harrison, Chester Arthur, Rutherford Hayes, and James Garfield.

June 24

TONIGHT'S CURE

Chopsticks. Half an hour before you go to bed, prepare your supper. Choose a meal that is not too acidic or fatty. A mixture of rice, lentils, and minced meat is easily digestible, or you can try a few boiled noodles with some tomatoes. Whatever you choose to eat, even if it is just a dry biscuit, try to eat it entirely with chopsticks. Then finish off the meal with an appropriate nightcap and get ready for bed.

TONIGHT'S TRIVIA

- The Queen of England is not allowed to enter the House of Commons.
- If you write a letter to nine different people one day, and each of them wrote to nine people the next day, and this process continued for ten days, approximately three-and-one-half billion people would receive letters, which is practically every person on earth!
- One of the first men to manufacture playing cards in America was Benjamin Franklin.
- The 18th Amendment (Prohibition) was never ratified by two states—Connecticut and Rhode Island.

June 25

TONIGHT'S CURE

Trees. Close your eyes and picture trees. Trees swaying gently in the night wind, trees silhouetted against a star-studded sky, and trees holding the warmth of the day in the delicious, heady, nighttime fragrance of the forest. Choose one tree you know well, one in your neighborhood or perhaps in your park. Start at the base of its trunk and work your way up with your eyes to the lower branches, up through the leaves, up to the very top of the tree. Now compile a list of trees from *A* to *Z*, *A* for ash, *B* for beech, *C* for cedar, and so on. When you've finished recall your first images and imagine the sound of the wind in the trees as you fall asleep.

- The Emperor Caligula gave his horse a golden drinking goblet from which the horse consumed wine.
- The nutritional value of the world's most widely eaten fish, herring, is the same as that of beefsteak.
- In July, 1765, a cow gave birth to a calf with two heads.
- Elephants live for more than a century.

June 26

TONIGHT'S CURE

Flying gull. Man has always wanted to fly unaided like a bird. But for the time being at least, the only way to succeed is in your imagination. If you concentrate hard, you can make it work however. Close your eyes and imagine that you are a gull flying through the air. Start at the seashore and launch yourself into the air flying up over the sea. Soar higher and higher and then spread your wings wide open and just glide peacefully along in the sun, floating on the wind without a care in the world.

TONIGHT'S TRIVIA

- The Bank at Monte Carlo has never been broken.
- A canon of Rheims, Peter de Riga, wrote a summary of the Bible in twenty-three sections, omitting in each section a particular letter of the alphabet.
- Eating ice cream makes you warmer.
- An ordinary conversation in the Arctic can be heard two miles away.

June 27

TONIGHT'S CURE

Short story time. If you find that your imagination is more active by night than by day, how about trying to write a short story for children as you lie awake. Imagine that you're writing for one of your own children, or the child of a friend. You can invent any characters you wish, and be as imaginative as you like, but you can't use any word containing the letter *E* and that's not easy!

TONIGHT'S TRIVIA

- If you freeze a bucket of seawater the ice will be free of salt.
- Nearly half the world's newspapers are published in North America.

- The Sargasso Sea is a sea without a shore.
- In 1811 an English blacksmith ate two pints of periwinkles, complete with shells, in twenty minutes to win a bet. He then died.

June 28

TONIGHT'S CURE

Be floored. Tonight get ready for bed. But instead of getting into bed as usual, take a pillow and a blanket or two and make yourself a little bed *on the floor*. Then get into this and attempt to go to sleep. However hard and uncomfortable it may appear, remain there for at least half an hour. Only after suffering for at least this long can you get into your own bed, which will now feel better than ever, and you should not have any problem falling asleep.

TONIGHT'S TRIVIA

- In 1752 Daniel McCurtley died At the age of eighty he married his fifth wife, who was only fifteen years old, by whom he had no fewer than fifteen children.
- The word *jeep* is derived from the letters *G.P.* which were stenciled on the U. S. Army's General Purpose car.
- Peter the Great of Russia could not read until he was fifteen.
- It is further from Honolulu to New York than it is from Honolulu to Japan.

June 29

TONIGHT'S CURE

Needle cure. Nearly every one of us has one article of clothing that needs repairing, or could at least be repaired if we put our mind to it. If you have a seam or hem coming undone, a button off, a small tear, a garment that requires lengthening or shortening, a sock that needs darning, then tonight is the night to get it done. If you have no sewing to do, then start some knitting, or even tapestry work. Many men find knitting and tapestry work very therapeutic, and relaxing. So get out your needles and get going!

TONIGHT'S TRIVIA

- Mustard will keep mice away.
- Once a tiger has tasted human flesh it becomes a man-eater for ever.
- A fish called the beaked chaetodon uses its nose as a gun to "shoot" insects with water.

• The chinook (warm wind) that occurs in Montana and Alberta can raise the air temperature by as much as 86° F in three minutes.

June 30

TONIGHT'S CURE

Sdrawkcab. Boring yourself to sleep often works, particularly if you have no interest in what you're doing. Try taking a favorite poem, novel, magazine article, or newspaper review to bed with you and read it backwards. It will not make any sense of course and you will find it so boring and difficult that you will not need to continue for long. When you've had enough, turn out the light, lie back on the bed, and start to recite your favorite poem, or the Lord's Prayer if you know nothing else by heart. But recite it backwards, starting with the last word first. You'll be asleep in no time.

TONIGHT'S TRIVIA

• People on earth never see more than one half of the moon because it moves around the earth with the same side facing us.
• Henry IV of France was married at the age of four to a three-year-old bride.
• Lead melts at 620° F.
• Two U.S. presidents, George Washington and Thomas Jefferson, had marijuana growing on their plantations.

July 1

TONIGHT'S CURE

Ice skating. Lie back and close your eyes. Imagine you are an ice skater on a very large deserted skating rink. The ice is smooth and clear. You are free to skate wherever and however you wish. Start by skating very fast, gliding along almost as if you were flying. Now spin round and round on the spot getting faster and faster and faster, until you feel completely exhausted.

TONIGHT'S TRIVIA

• The so-called four elements—earth, fire, air, and water—are all compounds.
• Nero did not fiddle while Rome burned—the fiddle had not yet been invented and besides, he was fifty miles away at the time.
• Tin melts at 446° F.
• In 1804 in Toulouse, France, a shower of frogs fell during a storm.

July 2

TONIGHT'S CURE

Bookworm. If you happen to be a committed bookworm, and as an insomniac this might just be the case, then this cure should not be too hard. All you have to do is compile an alphabetical list in your mind of all the books you have actually read. The first word of the title must begin with the letter of the alphabet. *The Farmer's Almanac* does not come under *F* for Farmer or *A* for Almanac, but *T* for The.

TONIGHT'S TRIVIA

• A sixteenth century prophet, Michael Nostradamus, who was born on this date, foretold, among others things: The French Revolution, Napoleon Bonaparte's exile, the rise of Adolf Hitler and Benito Mussolini; and the destruction of cities from the air.
• Railed tracks were used in Alsace mines since 1550.
• Passenger coaches were using sprung suspension by 1580.
• The first railroad in America, built in 1807, had wooden tracks.

July 3

TONIGHT'S CURE

Upside Down. Take a book, preferably one you have not read before. Turn the page upside down so that the top of the page will now be at the bottom. Looking at what is now the bottom of the page attempt to read the book, working your way from the bottom to the top of each page.

TONIGHT'S TRIVIA

• The speed limit for a tricycle in Vancouver is ten miles per hour.
• Frederick the Great used to have his veins opened in battle to calm his nerves.
• Napoleon Bonaparte was terrified of cats.
• If a kaleidoscope that contained twenty pieces was revolved to make 10 changes a minute, it would take 462,880,899,576 years and 360 days to exhaust the different combinations.

July 4

TONIGHT'S CURE

Midnight swim. Swimming can be a very strenuous activity, ideal for using up any excess energy. The weightlessness of the water will loosen strained muscles and generally refresh you so that you are totally relaxed and ready for bed. If you live near the sea, then there is nothing like a midnight swim, and having tried it I know it's true that the water is warmer at night. If you have a pool of your own then it will probably be more convenient to swim there, but if you haven't, pay a visit to a public pool during the evening, and enjoy a long, strenuous swim before coming home to bed.

TONIGHT'S TRIVIA

• If any whole number is decreased by the sum of its digits, the remainder is always exactly divisible by nine. Try it!

• In 1745 a flea was exhibited by a London watchmaker, tied by a chain of two hundred links, with a padlock and key, the whole weighing only one third of a grain.

• In 1883 a musical bed was manufactured in Paris. As soon as a person lay on it, a mechanism caused it to play tunes from famous operas. The price was a mere seventy thousand francs.

• President Coolidge was born on Independence Day 1872 and Presidents Adams, Jefferson, and Monroe all died on the Fourth of July. In fact Jefferson and Adams died at almost exactly the same minute on July 4, 1876. Monroe died five years later.

July 5
. . . .

TONIGHT'S CURE

Skeleton key to sleep. If you are frightened by skeletons, then substitute another cure. But if you are a medical student, or know your anatomy well, then you might find this cure therapeutic. Start at your toes with the tarsals, and name each bone in turn right up through your skeleton to the cranium. If you are a layman then simply say: the toe bones are connected to the heel bone, the heel bone is connected to the ankle bone, and on until you reach the skull.

TONIGHT'S TRIVIA

• Great Britain has more ghosts per square mile than any other country in the world.

• Mme. Marie Oliver, who admitted to bigamy in the sixteenth century, was sentenced to wearing two pairs of pants around her neck for the rest of her life.

• Philip II of Spain (1527–98) famed as being one of the most cowardly of people of all time, possessed the largest heart known to any man.

• With fewer than 6 percent of the people on earth the United States absorbs nearly 60 percent of the earth's resources.

July 6

TONIGHT'S CURE

Bedtime story. One very soothing cure for insomnia, and one which may take you back to childhood, is simply to get someone to read you a story. Choose a reader with a deep but pleasant sounding voice, not harsh or high-pitched. If there is no one available, get a friend to read you a story on a tape. Alternatively you can buy a prerecorded cassette, or read a story to yourself on tape.

TONIGHT'S TRIVIA

• Sophie Bunnen, the wife of a Pomeranian farmer, gave birth to eleven children in sixteen months. She had sextuplets and quintuplets.
• When the number 2,071,723 is multiplied by 5,363,222,357 the curious sum of 11,111,111,111,111,111 is produced.
• Petrus Placentius wrote a poem called *Pugna Porcorum* (The Battle of the Pigs) in which every verse began with the letter *P*.
• In 1973 a cat landed on a sidewalk in Montreal after falling from the twentieth floor. It limped away with one fractured pelvis.

July 7

TONIGHT'S CURE

Pugna Pocorum. Following Petrus Placentius' poem write a poem of your own in which every line begins with *P*. As you write the poem see how many words you can use beginning with this letter.

TONIGHT'S TRIVIA

• There were no aircraft carriers in World War I because they were not commissioned by the United States until 1922.
• In Scotland a chamber pot full of earth used to be given as a wedding present.
• A woman convicted of adultery during the reign of King Canute, by law, forfeited "both nose and ears."
• Queen Elizabeth I took a bath once a month, which amazed her courtiers who thought this was very fastidious.

July 8

TONIGHT'S CURE

Pillow stretch. Feeling a little restless tonight? Want to take some exercise without getting up? Then try this cure. Lie on your bed, on your back, on top of the covers. Place your hands on your hips and support your body with your elbows. Raise your legs into the air and lift your feet over your shoulders until they can grasp your pillow. Now lift it into the air and bring your feet down in front of you to drop the pillow at the end of the bed. Lie flat for a few minutes, then reverse the operation, replacing the pillow in its proper position. Do this three times and see if you're less worked up.

TONIGHT'S TRIVIA

• An Italian painter, Gugliemo Caccio, was the father of five nuns.
• In Peru there exists a bridge built by the Incas in 1350 that has been used for over five hundred years.
• The hand of St. Bartholomew is exhibited in the Abbey of St. Bartholomew in Wunstorf, Germany.
• U.S. submarines are named after fish, destroyers are named after naval heroes, cruisers are named after cities, and battleships are named after states.

July 9

TONIGHT'S CURE

Self massage. If you're desperate for a massage and there's no one around, there's only one solution—do it yourself. Take some baby oil or balm in your hands and massage it into your feet, in between the toes, on the soles, and around the ankles, Now work up your calves, rubbing and stroking in a soothing manner. Move upward to your knees and thighs, gently stroking and massaging. Massage every inch of your body, paying particular attention to your shoulders and neck. When you finish you should feel both relaxed and exhausted, if you massaged properly.

TONIGHT'S TRIVIA

• Peter the Great preserved the head of his executed mistress in a jar.
• There is no reference to a duck in the Old Testament.

- In Egypt a remedy for sterility used to be lying face upward under a passing train.
- A bottle of wine sold in London in 1960 was 420 years old.

July 10

TONIGHT'S CURE

Oatmeal gruel. Here's an old Scots cure to warm the cockles of your heart and send you soundly off to sleep. Take some porridge oats and make a thick porridge as directed on the packet. Then eat this very hot, with boiled milk and two tablespoons of honey, just before going to bed.

TONIGHT'S TRIVIA

- In the early 1800s people were still burned at the stake in the United States.
- Direct electrical current cannot be transmitted further than 1.9 miles.
- Prince Henry the Navigator, who never navigated a ship in his life, was given the title in spite of the fact that he had never even left Portugal.
- Almost one quarter of the male population of Tibet were Buddhist monks before the Chinese occupation in 1952.

July 11

TONIGHT'S CURE

Memoirs. One cure for insomnia favored by presidents and film stars is to think of a title for their memoirs. So why not think of a title for yours. Having thought of it try to visualize the title page coming off the press, bearing in mind that you have a print run of fifty thousand copies and you want to count each one.

TONIGHT'S TRIVIA

- The famous statue of Marcus Aurelius in Rome was used during the Middle Ages as a gallow.
- A natural rock formation in Ruhla, Germany, looks like a caveman.
- The albatross has a hooked beak and uses it like a pickax.
- The egg of the extinct Moa bird was seven inches long and five inches in diameter.

July 12

TONIGHT'S CURE

Can you see how.... Take a piece of paper and a pencil. Write down the longest sentence you can think of in which all the words are just three letters long. The record so far is a sentence of seventy four words, each of them three-lettered.

TONIGHT'S TRIVIA

• Male chauvinism is nothing new. A statue of Rameses II, built in 1225 B.C., depicts him over forty feet high, while the statue of his wife reaches only to his knee.

• The oldest-known painting of a European is on a wall in Crete and is five thousand years old.

• A town in Kentucky during the 1938 presidential election cast eighty-eight votes for Thomas Dewey and eighty-eight votes for Harry Truman.

• On July 12, 1961, the citizens of Shreveport, Louisiana, ran for their lives when the sky turned black and it rained green peaches.

July 13

TONIGHT'S CURE

Historical figure. Imagine you are a famous figure in history, perhaps someone you really admire. Maybe you're a queen like Cleopatra, or an explorer like Columbus, perhaps you're a past president, or a famous movie star of the silent screen. Try to imagine what life must have been like at that time. Picture the clothes you would have worn, what sort of home you would have had, and who your friends would have been. Try to imagine what every aspect of your "historical life" must have been like and if you could imagine every detail.

TONIGHT'S TRIVIA

• The hoatzin bird of northern South America has a head shaped like that of a small donkey.

• W. E. Gladstone, a past British prime minister, used to chew each mouthful of his food thirty times.

• In 1972 Napoleon Bonaparte's one-inch-long penis was put up for auction but failed to reach the reserve price.

• Only 16 percent of the able-bodied men in the American colonies actually took part in the Revolutionary War.

July 14

TONIGHT'S CURE

Ironing. Many people find that ironing is very therapeutic. So if you can't sleep, do all that ironing you've saved tonight and spend the time that you would have been ironing doing something else. Instead of going to bed at your usual time, start ironing. As you smooth out each garment, feel that you are smoothing over all your troubles and cares. Once you've finished the work there will be great satisfaction in having gotten one more job out of the way and you'll be able to relax knowing that everything is clean and fresh for tomorrow.

TONIGHT'S TRIVIA

- Champagne was originally invented by a monk.
- To lose one pound of fat you have to walk thirty-four miles.
- A female mosquito can produce 150 million offspring in one year.
- One American folk hero was born and another died on this date. On July 14, 1925, Woody Guthrie was born in Ohemah, Oklahoma, while on July 14, 1881, Pat Garrett shot the outlaw Billy the Kid.

July 15

TONIGHT'S CURE

Shower massage. Today is St. Swithin's Day, the day associated with rain. So it's only right that tonight's cure should be associated with rain too. No, you don't go into the yard and stand in a thunderstorm, you go into the shower instead. Turn it on full blast so it hits your body with all its force. Now place each part of your body under the shower in turn and let the water massage that particular part. If you can, lie down in the shower and raise your legs into the air so that the water massages the soles of your feet and runs all over your body. Close your eyes and imagine that you are in fact standing in a warm tropical downpour. Listen to the sound of the water washing away your cares. Then dry yourself quickly and go straight to bed.

TONIGHT'S TRIVIA

- Overweight schoolchildren quite frequently eat less than their slimmer contemporaries.

- Muscles only work by pulling, they never push.
- Women's ears were thought to be erogenous zones during the Middle Ages and had to be covered.
- The world's tallest man, Robert Wadlow of Monistree, Michigan, died on July 15, 1960. He stood 8 feet 11.1 inches. On the same day in 1883 the world's shortest man, Charles ("General Tom Thumb") Stratton also died. He was almost exactly double Wadlow's age, but was only 3-feet 4-inches tall.

July 16

TONIGHT'S CURE

Space shuttle. Ever felt like floating above it all, literally, without a care in the world? Then imagine you are an astronaut in space. Pretend that you are warmly and safely fitted into your space suit and are about to walk into space for the first time. Visualize the complete darkness around you. Feel your utter weightlessness as you float out of the hatch into this great void. And now experience the pleasure of the lack of gravity and the absence of worldly worries.

TONIGHT'S TRIVIA

- As late as 1675, griffins were still listed among the animals that were saved in Noah's ark.
- Einstein did not believe in using shaving cream.
- George Washington's dentist pioneered the first dentist's drill using his mother's spinning wheel.
- Originally an abracadabra was a charm used to cure hay fever.

July 17

TONIGHT'S CURE

Adam's apple. Whether you are an Adam or an Eve this remedy should have the same effect. Take a very large apple to bed with you. Sit in bed; look at the apple, feel it, touch it, smell it. Use all your senses on this one object. Lay it down for a minute. Imagine the apple in your mind, picture it, feel it, smell it. After four to five minutes pick up the apple again and eat it very slowly. Chew each bite carefully and enjoy every mouthful and drop of juice.

TONIGHT'S TRIVIA

- In 1913 a very rare Roman coin was found buried in Illinois.

- Lamprey eels build nests of stone four feet high at the bottom of the sea. Male and female eels carry the stones together.
- There is a natural rock formation in Czechoslovakia which looks like a ruined castle.
- The Ainu women of Japan always cover their mouths when speaking to a man.

July 18

TONIGHT'S CURE

Card house. Tonight try your hand at a manual cure for insomnia. Take a large tray and a pack of cards to bed with you. Sit up straight in bed, place the tray on your lap, and start to build a card house on the tray. You will need to keep very still and it will take great concentration if you are going to succeed. But there is a great sense of satisfaction that comes when you build the house, blow it down, and then turn out the light and go to sleep.

TONIGHT'S TRIVIA

- John Wilson of Port Credit, Ontario, built a house of cards 39 stories high, using 1,240 playing cards.
- Fans found in the tomb of Tutankhamun still had ostrich feathers which were intact after three thousand years.
- Shoes worn by Australian aborigines have emu-feather soles so they leave no footprints.
- The Capitol in Wisconsin has the largest granite dome of any building in the United States.

July 19

TONIGHT'S CURE

Witch hazel. One of the oldest cures for insomnia is said to be witch hazel, claimed to have soporific qualities. To try this cure, simply soak some cotton in witch hazel, place two cotton pads on your eyelids and keep them in place with a bandage tied around your head. Then lie back and let the witch hazel get to work.

TONIGHT'S TRIVIA

- Chinese tumble dolls were originally made in the image of Buddha to prove that Buddha could not fall.
- In 1908 a mass of iron weighing forty thousand tons fell from the sky in Siberia.

- *Don Quixote* has been translated into more languages than any other book, excluding the Bible.
- Humble pie has nothing to do with humility; cheap cuts of meat were once called *umbles.*

July 20

TONIGHT'S CURE

Open wide. Going to sleep normally requires you to close your eyes, but in this case you have to try to keep them as wide open as you can. Sit up in bed with the lights turned out and open your eyes as wide as you can, trying to hold them open without blinking. It won't be long before your eyes start to feel unbearably heavy and you fall asleep.

TONIGHT'S TRIVIA

- Charles Robert Lockheart, state treasurer of Texas in 1930, was a midget.
- In colonial America shoes were made to be worn on either foot.
- The first film star to become famous was named Florence Lawrence.
- The sword-bill hummingbird has a beak longer than its body.

July 21

TONIGHT'S CURE

Pseudonyms. With tonight's cure you can leave your own worries and anxieties behind and adopt a comforting "alter ego." Imagine that you have written what will be a best-selling novel, but do not want your friends and co-workers to know that you are going to become a multimillionaire. Try to select a pseudonym for yourself, a name you really like and feels comfortable. Imagine what it looks like in print. Say it over and over again to yourself.

TONIGHT'S TRIVIA

- Arabic was not spoken in Egypt until the seventeenth century.
- The Old Faithful geyser in Yellowstone National Park shoots boiling water into the air every hour.
- In conversation *I* is the most frequently used word.
- On July 21, 1873, the first railroad robbery took place near Adair, Iowa, when the James-Younger gang held up a train. On the same date, ninety-six years later, man first walked on the moon's surface.

July 22

TONIGHT'S CURE

Just face it. The major muscles that relax when you are asleep are your facial muscles, which is why your mouth sometimes hangs open and your eyelids are only very lightly closed. In order to sleep try to let every muscle in your face relax. Stretch your mouth into a big grin, and let it relax. Wrinkle up your nose, and let it relax. Raise your eyebrows as high as they will go, and let them relax. Move your scalp backwards and forwards, and then let it relax. Finally screw up your entire face as tightly as you can, and let it all relax. Repeat this five times and then lie back on the pillow with your eyes shut ready for sleep.

TONIGHT'S TRIVIA

• The office of executioner in France was hereditary, which explains why Charles Sanson inherited the post of chief executioner in 1726—at the age of seven.
• The orchid gets its name from the Greek word for testicles.
• Leo Tolstoy, the Russian novelist whose heroine Anna Karenina died in a railway station, ironically died in a railway station himself.
• Robert E. Lee had been offered the command of the Union Army before he took up his post with the Confederacy.

July 23

TONIGHT'S CURE

Hot mustard. One of history's most popular, and most effective, ways of easing tension is a hot mustard bath. This is simple to prepare and delightful to use. Just before going to bed, fill a bowl with hot, but not boiling, water. Add three tablespoons of mustard powder to the water and stir it around. Then put your feet into the bowl and steep them for ten to fifteen minutes in the warm, relaxing bath, before drying them quickly and hopping straight into bed.

TONIGHT'S TRIVIA

• Arthur E. Gehrke of Watertown, hibernated each winter by sleeping from Thanksgiving to Easter each year for over twenty-three years.
• At every moment there are at least two thousand thunderstorms taking place on the earth's surface.

- Russia is the greatest consumer of perfume in the world.
- The queen that appears on English playing cards represents that of Henry VII's wife, Elizabeth of York.

July 24

TONIGHT'S CURE

Through the mattress. Lying on your bed with the light out, lie on your back, preferably with one pillow. Let your limbs relax completely and feel your mattress becoming softer and softer. Feel yourself sinking down into the mattress until you almost feel as if you are lying on a cloud. Now let your mattress completely engulf you as you drift off to sleep.

TONIGHT'S TRIVIA

- The great white shark is the only creature in the world that has no natural enemies.
- The worst tornado ever recorded hurtled over Texas at a speed of 290.33 miles per hour.
- One ice that does not melt is dry ice—it evaporates.
- Lions are only 10 percent successful in catching their prey.

July 25

TONIGHT'S CURE

Cut down. If you consistently spend two or three hours awake each night it could mean that you are trying to get too much sleep. It is pure fallacy to think that everyone needs eight hours of sleep. Some people only *need* four or five hours. Napoleon needed very little and philosopher R. Buckminster Fuller slept for just four hours a day, taking half an hour every three hours. So try and cut down on the length of time you spend in bed and you may find that you do in fact sleep better.

TONIGHT'S TRIVIA

- St. Augustus of Hippo is the patron saint of brewers.
- Of the Christmas cards bought today, 20 percent are in aid of charity.
- Nine out of ten Indian girls are married before they are twenty years old.
- Locusts take seventeen years to reach adulthood.

July 26

TONIGHT'S CURE

Two under blankets. Could your bedding be keeping you awake? Tonight put two blankets underneath your bottom sheet and lie on those, covering yourself very loosely. You will find that this will make you much more comfortable.

TONIGHT'S TRIVIA

• Every verse of Psalm 136 ends with the same words, *"For his steadfast love endures for ever."*
• Bachelors have a much higher suicide rate than married men.
• The first airplanes were modeled on box kites.
• In Luxembourg, two and one-half times more beer than wine is consumed.

July 27

TONIGHT'S CURE

Cow's remedy. This cure is the product of cows—milk! Take a whole pint of ice-cold milk to bed with you. Make sure that it is very cold, taken straight from the refrigerator. Once you're in bed, sip it slowly, sitting upright. Try and drink the whole pint. Then lie back on your pillows until you feel comfortable and relaxed. Close your eyes and fall asleep.

TONIGHT'S TRIVIA

• Carriages in the early nineteenth century were subject to a federal tax.
• When the American crew of Apollo X reentered the earth's atmosphere in 1969, they were traveling at 24,790.8 miles per hour—faster than any man had ever traveled before.
• In Brisbane, Australia, a seventeen-year-old flamenco dancer achieved a tap rate of one thousand heel taps per minute.
• Richard Wagner was Franz Liszt's son-in-law.

July 28

TONIGHT'S CURE

Camp bed. Sometimes a change of bed can make you appreciate your own bed all the more. Tonight might be a good time to try out this idea. Set up a camp bed in the room next to yours, or even in the living room, anywhere but in your own bedroom. Spend the first hour of the night sleeping on this bed, and then move back to your own bed—unless of course you find the camp bed more comfortable and you decide to remain there all night.

TONIGHT'S TRIVIA

• Surveys show that professors who smoke are twice as likely to write books as those who do not smoke.
• The silkworm is a caterpillar.
• The first pilot to fly solo in Australia was the famous escapologist, Harry Houdini.
• Ferrets can catch a cold just like humans.

July 29

TONIGHT'S CURE

Cloud nine. Can you imagine what it would be like to have your spirit drifting among the clouds? Lie back on your bed in your most comfortable position and see if you can. Make sure that you are warm. Let all your muscles relax. Close your eyes. Feel yourself raise into the air, which is similar to the feeling you have when you're fainting, and then drift up until you reach the clouds. Picture what it would be like looking down from the fluffy white clouds and float away to peaceful oblivion.

TONIGHT'S TRIVIA

• In 1976, 150 million bottles of Coca-Cola were bought daily.
• A ram adds an additional spiral section to its horns annually.
• There are two thousand varieties of German sausage.
• The murder rate in medieval times was twenty-six times greater than it is today.

July 30

TONIGHT'S CURE

On the top. Tonight when it is time for bed, go through the usual nightly routine of cleaning your teeth, putting the cat out, listening to the late news, etc. But when you turn in do not remove your clothes or get under the covers. Simply lie on the top of the bed, fully dressed, reading a magazine or a book. Only when you begin to feel really sleepy should you remove your clothes and get into bed to fall asleep.

TONIGHT'S TRIVIA

• A caterpillar has over two thousand muscles in its body.

• The English scientist, Sir Isaac Newton, wrote over one-hundred thousand pages of notes on astrology and the occult.

• During World War II the Oscar Award was made out of wood to conserve valuable metal.

• Patents for gambling machines cannot be taken out in the United States.

July 31

TONIGHT'S CURE

Office prescription. One of the most frequent causes of insomnia is anxiety about work. Sometimes actively thinking about a place of work can help you sleep. Try it. Visualize an office, your own if you have one. Walk in and look around. Try to list every piece of equipment you see there in alphabetical order, starting with *A* for accounts file, *B* for blind on the window, and continue until you reach *Z*. If you are still awake, however, try listing the various departments of an office in alphabetical order, and see how many departments you can allocate to each letter.

TONIGHT'S TRIVIA

• Only the male canary sings.

• Madame de Pompadour of France was the first person to own a pet goldfish.

• Many breeds of tropical fish could survive in an aquarium filled with human blood.

• The only eggs that you can spin are hard boiled eggs.

August 1

TONIGHT'S CURE

Goldfish. Madame de Pompadour may have been the first to own a pet fish, but they are now very popular and it is possible that you may have your own tropical fish at home. If you don't have any, a couple of goldfish are worth investing in to help cure your insomnia. Place the bowl or tank beside your bed and watch the fish swimming around at night. This has a wonderfully hypnotic and soporific effect. Try to imagine yourself as a goldfish. Think how few worries they have, how easy life is for them. Watch them closely for at least ten minutes, then turn off the light and imagine that you are swimming around in the bowl. That should help you quickly fall asleep.

TONIGHT'S TRIVIA

- The British spend twice as much on pet food as they spend on baby food.
- Chameleons found in Burma are the only ones that have horns.
- The first dry martini was concocted in 1860.
- If you magnified a glass of water to the size of the earth the molecules would appear as big as oranges.

August 2

TONIGHT'S CURE

Skipping. Strenuous physical exercise just before you get into bed can often tire you sufficiently to send you off to sleep. Skipping is particularly effective and is easy to do in the bedroom. Take a child's jump rope, or a long cord from your robe, and get undressed and ready for bed. Just before getting in, take your rope and start skipping around the bedroom. Skip for five to ten minutes, depending upon how fit you are. Then get into bed, relax, and fall into a deep sleep.

TONIGHT'S TRIVIA

- The redwood tree has a fireproof bark.
- Crushed strawberries will relieve sunburn.
- Wild Bill Hickok was shot dead in a saloon in Deadwood, South Dakota, on August 2, 1876. On the same date in 1923 President Warren G. Harding died under mysterious circumstances in San Francisco. Facing the possibility of impeachment and public disgrace many believed that Harding had taken his own life. However, the doctors attending him could not agree on a cause of death, and his wife refused to allow an autopsy, which pointed the finger of blame toward her.
- As they grow older male monkeys lose the hair on their heads just as men do.

August 3

TONIGHT'S CURE

Stomach massage. If you've eaten a rich meal before going to bed, this might be keeping you awake. If it is, try this cure. Lie on your back, draw your knees upward, and massage your stomach, first with your right hand, then with your left. Continue to do this for five to ten minutes. This will get rid of any excess gas that may have built up in your body which may be keeping you awake.

TONIGHT'S TRIVIA

• A thirty-two-year-old Milwaukee rabbi once skipped nonstop for four hours and ten minutes.
• Lake Baskunchak, in Russia, has enough salt in it to supply the world for over two thousand years.
• Domestic cats spend only one-third of their lives awake. (Insomnia is not one of their chief problems.)
• Over half the people bitten by poisonous snakes in the United States who are not treated still manage to survive.

August 4

TONIGHT'S CURE

Knock knees. Concentrating on the parts of your body you don't normally see might seem a strange way of sending yourself to sleep, but it works in some instances. This is what you do. Lie in bed in a comfortable position. Close your eyes and focus your attention on your knees. No matter what other thoughts enter your mind, dismiss them immediately and just think of your knees. You'll find it very difficult to do and it may take you a couple of nights to perfect, but it really is worth it if you can succeed.

TONIGHT'S TRIVIA

• In the late seventeenth century, tea was pronounced *tay*.
• Surgeons in ancient Egypt had their hands cut off if their patients died.
• Abraham Lincoln was the first U. S. president to be assassinated.
• The largest airport in the world is in Forth Worth, Texas, covering an area greater than six and a half thousand football fields.

August 5

TONIGHT'S CURE

Fantasize. Doctors and psychologists claim that there is nothing medically or morally harmful about erotic thoughts, and to many people erotic fantasies are a natural and enjoyable way of getting to sleep. It may be a natural occupation for you anyway! But if it's not, try imagining that you are Casanova or Cleopatra, a superstud or a seductress, and that your bedroom is filled with hundreds of naked, nubile young women and men. Then really let your imagination rip.

TONIGHT'S TRIVIA

• Pope Paul IV was so horrified by naked figures painted by Michelangelo in *The Last Judgement* that another artist was commissioned to add the clothes!

• Debauchees do not wear themselves out and die young; Casanova was seventy-three when he died and Catherine the Great was sixty-seven.

• The first striptease took place in Paris, in 1893, and caused a riot.

• Socialist Eugene Debs, who received 920,000 votes in his bid for the presidency in 1920, conducted his whole campaign while in jail.

August 6

TONIGHT'S CURE

White House. Power, total power—how many of us dream of it and how many of us ever attain it? Well, tonight's your chance. Imagine that you are living in the White House, that you are the President or America's First Lady, but with absolutely no responsibility whatsoever. Imagine that you have a free hand and can simply enjoy yourself. Picture each of the rooms in the house and what you would do with them in such a position. What other privileges would your new-found status afford you, and how would you use them to their best advantage?

TONIGHT'S TRIVIA

• The mangrove tree grows in salt water.

• More than one-hundred million comets revolve around the sun.

• The multiple name for a group of barrage balloons is "balloon barrage."

• The cheer Hip, Hip, Hooray originated from the time of the conquest of Jerusalem by the Saracens.

August 7

TONIGHT'S CURE

Play reading. Those quiet night hours when everyone else is sleeping could be your one chance to exercise your dramatic flair, free from embarrassment and out of the public eye. Choose a favorite play and take it to bed with you tonight. Read the play aloud, reading each of the character's parts yourself, and giving each character a different and identifiable voice. Read at least the first act aloud and enjoy your very own late night drama, uninhibited and uninterrupted. You never know, it may set you dreaming completely new dreams.

TONIGHT'S TRIVIA

• The French actress Sarah Bernhardt enjoyed over one thousand lovers during her lifetime, and frequently slept in a coffin.
• William Shakespeare had red hair.
• Sir Noel Coward wrote one of his most successful comedies, *Hay Fever,* in three days.
• Only seven of Sophocles' 123 plays survived.

August 8

TONIGHT'S CURE

Animal magic. Most people tend to keep pets out of their bedroom for reasons of hygiene, although there is no reason why a cat or dog should be less hygienic during the night than during the daytime. People who do allow their dogs to sleep in their bedrooms, however, rarely suffer from insomnia. So if you have a cat or dog, allow his or her basket, or bed, in your room tonight. You could even let him sleep at the foot of your bed—unless you have a St. Bernard or Great Dane of course! The presence and warmth of another living creature in the room will give you a sense of security and comfort.

TONIGHT'S TRIVIA

• Piano woods are generally made from the wood of hornbeam trees.
• Solar energy has been used to power toys since 1615.
• St. Simeon the Younger spent the last forty-five years of his life sitting on top of a pole.
• A French actor, Pierre Messie, could make his hair stand on end at will.

August 9

TONIGHT'S CURE

White room. You may have already experienced the white sheet cure. If you have this one may strike a chord of interest. Close your eyes and imagine that you are in a white room. The walls are white. The floor is white. The ceiling is white. There is no furniture in the room. There are no windows. There are no doors. The room is completely square and white. You are lying in the middle of a mat-white robe, unbroken by any color and any features. Close your eyes on this monotonous scene and fall asleep.

TONIGHT'S TRIVIA

• Robert Graves wrote some of his most passionate and sensual love poetry when he was over sixty.
• The first edition of the *Encyclopaedia Brittanica* gave actual factual evidence about Noah's Ark.
• The Bible says that a serpent stings with its tail; it was Shakespeare who introduced the belief that a snake's forked tongue could sting.
• Upon the death of Adlai Stevenson, Richard Nixon remarked: "In eloquence of expression, he had no peers and very few equals."

August 10

TONIGHT'S CURE

Alphabetical animals. Imagine you are strolling around a zoo. Look into each of the pens and list the animals you see in alphabetical order, beginning with *A* for aardvark, *B* for buffalo, *C* for chimpanzee, *D* for dolphin, through *Z* for zebra. Then when you reach *Z,* say the list in reverse order until you reach *A* again.

TONIGHT'S TRIVIA

• Beetles outnumber any other living creature on earth.
• An elephant has one hundred pounds of brain for every one thousand pounds of its body weight.
• Until 1789 lions were used to guard the Tower of London.
• A deer sheds its antlers every year and grows new ones.

August 11

TONIGHT'S CURE

Deaths in office. Since 1840 every U. S. president elected in a year ending with a zero has died in office (except for President Reagan). John F. Kennedy was the most recent. See if you can list all the presidents who were elected in a year ending with a zero.

TONIGHT'S TRIVIA

- Two hills near Casteldelci, Italy, are naturally shaped like pyramids.
- In 1910 President William Taft initiated the presidential custom of pitching the first ball in a baseball game.
- President John Tyler was so disliked by Congress that it would not allocate funds to replace patched carpeting and tattered drapes in the White House.
- Dolphins sleep with one eye open.

August 12

TONIGHT'S CURE

Washington. Lie in bed with the light out if you have a good memory and are in the habit of solving crosswords in your head. If you can't do that, keep the light on and use a sheet of paper. Now think of the word *Washington*. Repeat it slowly to yourself several times before trying to make as many words out of it as you can. All the words have to contains three or more letters, and you can only use the ten letters that the word contains. The final rule is that you can't repeat any of the letters more than once. Have a go tonight. It'll soon send you off to sleep.

TONIGHT'S TRIVIA

- President Theodore Roosevelt used a hollowed-out rhinocerous foot as an inkwell.
- On August, 12, 1676, the Indian war ended in New England. On the same date in 1898 the United States formally annexed Hawaii.
- The area of the United States covered by highway is equal to the area of the state of West Virginia.
- The Virgin Mary has appeared on the front cover of *Time* magazine more than any other woman.

August 13

TONIGHT'S CURE

Talk aloud therapy. Don't bottle your worries up inside you any longer. When you get into bed tonight sit up when you turn off the light and start listing aloud all those aggravating little things and major things that are worrying you. However small and trivial they may seem, they must be weighing heavily on your mind and it is certainly best to get them off your chest now. You can talk to your God, to Buddha, to whomever you may believe in; talk to the wall if you believe in nothing. Say "I am worried about how I am going to pay my electricity bill; I hate Josh Lupino at work; one of my teeth aches slightly but I hate visiting the dentist; I think my daughter is having an affair with the minister; I can't stand the paintwork in mother's lounge; I can't afford the new shoes I want." Just keep on talking until you fall asleep.

TONIGHT'S TRIVIA

• Every bucket of seawater contains two cups of dissolved minerals.
• The first woman to take her seat in the British House of Commons was Viscountess Astor, an American.
• The Smithsonian Institution was founded by a man who never once set foot in the United States—James Smithson, an English scientist.
• A survey of U.S. physicians taken in 1977 showed that fewer than 9 percent were women.

August 14

TONIGHT'S CURE

Colors. Use the darkness of your bedroom tonight to let your mind wander over a rainbow. Close your eyes and start to think of the names of all the colors you've ever seen. Start with the obvious ones—red, blue, green yellow—and then branch out to violet, lemon, crimson, mauve, steel grey, skyblue, pale pink, and all the myriad colors that exist in nature. Once you've listed all the colors you can think of, close your eyes very tightly and visualize each of them in turn. What associations do they have? Do your days of the week have colors? If they do, why? Is it some distant childhood memory? Why are some colors your favorites? Why can't you stand others? Walk a rainbow of memories tonight before you sleep.

TONIGHT'S TRIVIA

• Apes, guinea pigs, and man are the only animals not capable of producing vitamin C in their bodies.
• One of the greatest dilemmas faced by artists throughout history was whether or not they should paint Adam and Eve with navels.
• On the average we lose eleven ounces while we sleep.
• It takes seventeen muscles to smile and forty-three to frown.

August 15

TONIGHT'S CURE

Huggy huggy. Remember how your Teddy used to help you sleep all those years ago? Remember the security and comfort you got from large, fluffy toys when you were little? Perhaps you need that now. Get yourself a very large toy; a big fluffy dog, a large teddy bear, a stuffed elephant, absolutely anything that is large and soft and warm. Whatever you choose, take it to bed with you, hugging it tightly in your arms. Imagine that your comforter is lonely too and that it needs you just as much. Give each other mutual protection tonight and perhaps you'll both sleep soundly.

TONIGHT'S TRIVIA

• It is impossible to see a gaggle of geese flying. Once in the air they become a skein.
• The rate of acceleration of the flea when it jumps is nearly thirty times greater than the speed at which a human being blacks out.
• Cleopatra's Needle in London has little to with Cleopatra. It was erected almost fifteen hundred years before she was born.
• Orval Overall, Eli Grba, Tony Suck, Coot Veal, Prince Oana, Malachi Kittredge, and Yats Wuestling were all major-league baseball stars.

August 16

TONIGHT'S CURE

Artist's model. Imagine tonight that you are posing to have your portrait painted by the world's leading portrait painter. The artist wants you to pose reclining so get yourself into a comfortable reclining position, one in which you will be able to remain for some time without getting stiff. Once you're in position you must remain like that without moving. You can of course fall asleep. In fact the painter encourages you to close your eyes.

TONIGHT'S TRIVIA

• Blood takes only one minute to be pumped around the body by your heart.
• In 1888, 246 people were killed by hailstones in India.
• Wolfgang Mozart died in 1791, convinced he was being poisoned by Italians.
• The Battle of Bennington, Vermont, and the Battle of Camden,

South Carolina, were fought on August 16, 1777 and 1780 respectively.

August 17

TONIGHT'S CURE

Skip a night. If you really feel in need of a good sleep, and this is not a cure to be repeated very often, try going one complete night without any sleep at all. Plan it very carefully so that you can keep yourself fully occupied. Choose a night when there are programs that you want to watch on TV until late into the night. Make it a night when you don't have to work the next day. Start cooking your last meal in the early hours of the night. Make it a meal that takes a lot of preparation, and sit and enjoy it. This could occupy two hours of the night. Do some work first, even if it is only housework. Read some books. Then sit at a window, or better still, go for a walk and experience the pleasure of watching the dawn come up and hearing the early-morning sounds. When you reach your normal waking time in the morning you will probably feel no ill effects at all, but tomorrow night you will sleep like a log. Take this cure no more than once every three months though—you'll value its effect all the more!

TONIGHT'S TRIVIA

• The Tuatora, found in New Zealand, has a family history 180 million years old and is one of the few surviving dinosaurs.
• Johann von Goethe wrote a story in seven languages when he was ten.
• A migrating English swallow takes one month to reach its wintering grounds in Africa.
• Davy Crockett was born in Hawkins County, Tennessee, on August 17, 1786, and Mae West shared his birthday when she was born in Brooklyn, in 1892.

August 18

TONIGHT'S CURE

At a stroke. Perhaps you've sent your kids to sleep by gently stroking their brows? Perhaps you were sent to sleep in this way when you were a kid? It's one of the most soothing ways to end a care-worn day, as you'll find if you get someone to stroke your forehead very gently as you lie in bed tonight. All that is required is a very light stroke with the fingertips moving from right to left, or from left to right, but constantly stroking in the same direction. Close your eyes and you'll be out like a light.

TONIGHT'S TRIVIA

• In Tibet it is a gesture of respect to stick your tongue out at your guests.
• Bees and rabbits originated in Australia.
• Before driver's licenses became legal a six-year-old British child was discovered riding a motorcycle.
• Three U. S. presidents were born in Norfolk County, Massachusetts: John Adams, John Quincy Adams, and John F. Kennedy.

August 19

TONIGHT'S CURE

Book head. Here's a cure for insomnia that should help improve your deportment as well as sending you to sleep. When you get into bed tonight sit up straight, check that your spine is straight, and then turn out the light. Now take a paperback book, and in the dark, balance it on top of your head. Keep your eyes looking straight out into the dark and balance the book for as long as you can. When it falls off you'll probably be ready for sleep.

TONIGHT'S TRIVIA

• Caviar is 30 percent protein.
• One campaign against alcoholism in Australia had to be disbanded due to lack of support.
• In 1883 a Chinese priest decided to grow his fingernails. By 1910 they were nearly twenty-three inches long.
• In the Basque language the word *Jingo* means God.

August 20

TONIGHT'S CURE

Count your blessings. As you lie awake tonight, put out of your mind all the things that are wrong in your life, all the problems that may exist, the things you have been mistaken over and would like to improve. Instead, start to count the good things in your life, the things you have to be thankful for; your family, your eyesight, your power of speech, your ability to read, your hearing, your love, your talents, your material possessions, the fact that you have your health and strength. List these blessings in your mind and you'll soon see that there is always somebody somewhere who is *much* worse off than you are.

• In the Puamo Islands of the Eastern Pacific, the natives decorate their ankles and shoulders with the hair of their departed relatives when performing ritual dances.
• There are six languages in North America which have just one surviving speaker.
• In 1809 one Captain Barclay succeeded in walking one thousand miles in one thousand hours.
• The oil in which sardines are packed is more expensive than the sardines themselves.

August 21

TONIGHT'S CURE

Rhythmical words. Children and young animals can often be sent to sleep with an artificial heartbeat, so there's no reason why a rhythmical beat shouldn't have the same effect on you, if you're willing to give it a try. Put a loud ticking clock beside your bed before you turn out the light and then listen to its steady tick as you lie in the dark—tick tock tick tock. Now listen to the clock changing rhythm in your mind, so that you hear it going tick tock tock, tick tock tock. Finally put words to whichever rhythm you choose to hear: "I can sleep, I can sleep..." or "I am tired, I am tired...." Match the rhythm of the ticking to the rhythm of your thoughts and let the two lull you to sleep.

TONIGHT'S TRIVIA

• George Washington used dentures made of wood and ivory.
• Francois Voltaire used to drink fifty cups of coffee a day.
• The Earl of Sterling once rented the whole of Canada for one penny a year.
• A decree passed in the African state of Guinea, in 1976, made military service compulsory for boys aged seven to fourteen.

August 22

TONIGHT'S CURE

Universal cure. As you lie awake tonight think how small and insignificant your worries are in relation to the rest of the universe, and how trivial and silly they all must seem to the world outside. Remember that, whatever your major problem is, *all* *things pass in time.* I was told that years ago by a marvelous eighty-four-year-old lady who never worried about a thing, and she was right. Thinking about the world and the universe will put your own small personal problems back into perspective.

TONIGHT'S TRIVIA

• In eighteenth century England ladies wore beauty patches on their faces that also indicated which political party they supported.
• The first U. S. law passed against lynching made the accused liable to four years in prison.
• One of the earliest airships looked like a canoe supported by balloons.
• In the Middle East state of Oman it was illegal to play drums until 1970.

August 23

TONIGHT'S CURE

Stroll or cure. If tonight is fine, and we sincerely hope it is, put on a light coat and set out on a brisk walk at your normal bedtime. Aim to walk *at least* one mile, preferably longer if you can. Take your sleeping partner or your dog with you, if you do not want to walk alone, and (if you are worried about being attacked) a large umbrella or stick. Enjoy the cool night air and the peace that only nighttime brings.

TONIGHT'S TRIVIA

• In 1966 the River Arno flooded in Florence causing over $100 million worth of damage to art treasures.
• Glaciers cover 10 percent of the earth.
• The first and last letters of each continents' name are alike.
• The Marine Corps were originally established as a unit of the British army stationed in the American colonies.

August 24

TONIGHT'S CURE

Last movie. Think back to the very last movie you saw. Do you remember the plot? Can you recall the music? Try to visualize the opening credits and the opening scene. From there try to relive the entire film in your mind. Remember each of the characters. Remember the dialogue. Take on the role of one of the characters if you like and picture yourself up on the screen acting out whichever part you choose.

TONIGHT'S TRIVIA

• A brush for applying varnish will give one hundred times more wear than one used for paint.
• In the seventeenth century it was illegal to celebrate Christmas in Massachusetts.
• The world's most popular hobby is stamp collecting.
• There is a lake on the Indonesian Island of Java that blows bubbles into the air.

August 25

TONIGHT'S CURE

Party time. Do you want to exhaust yourself and enjoy it at the same time? Here's a fun way of going about it—throw a party. You can either make it a lavish dinner party with no fewer than eight people, or have a wine and cheese party with a minimum of twenty guests. Whichever you choose it will make you very popular with your friends; you'll be able to repay hospitality, it will give you something to put your mind to and look forward to, and the preparation and organization involved will give you a good night's sleep for several nights before the party.

TONIGHT'S TRIVIA

• In 1904 an American razor company sold 12,400,000 razor blades.
• Lawn tennis originated from a game played by eleventh century monks.
• The telephone developed as a result of hearing-aid research.
• Albert Einstein did not speak until he was four years old.

August 26

TONIGHT'S CURE

Family album. Tonight, at last, you've got a chance to get out your family album and all those old photographs, even old holiday snapshots. Can you identify all the people on the photographs? Do you remember all the places and dates surrounding the pictures? Let your mind wander through the reminiscences recalled by your trip down memory lane. What were your worries and problems then? Don't they seem trivial now? Won't your present ones soon be trivial too?

TONIGHT'S TRIVIA

- The Great Pyramid of Cheops is the largest sun dial in the world.
- The word *tycoon* entered our language from the Chinese.
- Goldfish left in a dark room for a long time will turn white.
- A sea urchin walks on the ends of its teeth.

August 27

TONIGHT'S CURE

Sea bed. Imagine that you have the power to breathe under water without the aid of a diving suit and oxygen. Imagine also that it is light on the sea bed, and you can look around without needing artificial light. Once you've reached the ocean floor sense the weightlessness and total support of the water. Visualize the beauty of the strange fish and colorful plants that you see growing in abundance all around you. Now walk toward an enormous shell in front of you. It's large enough for you to crawl inside, so go in and curl up, warm and comfortable, and slowly fall into a silent, weightless sleep.

TONIGHT'S TRIVIA

- The cashew nut belongs to the poison ivy family.
- The only insect to produce food eaten by man is the bee.
- In Kenya elephants bathe in a mud which, when it dries, turns pink on their skins, literally turning them into pink elephants.
- On August 27, 1883, the island of Krakatoa exploded with such force that the blast was heard three thousand miles away, rocks were blown thirty-four miles through the air, and the subsequent tidal waves traveled seventy-five hundred miles to Cape Horn.

August 28

TONIGHT'S CURE

Birthday cards. Do you ever lie awake agonizing over a birthday that you've forgotten. Perhaps that's the reason you can't sleep tonight. Whatever the cause of your insomnia though, start to make a list in your mind of every single person to whom you send a birthday card. Start in January and work through to December, giving the exact date of the birthday in question. Having done that, and today will be somebody's birthday somewhere, start on January 1 and work through every day trying to think of a person who was born on that particular day. See if you can think of at least 365 birthdays before you fall asleep. If you can't, continue your list the next time you're lying awake and unable to sleep.

TONIGHT'S TRIVIA

• Pope Benedict IX became Pope at the age of eleven.

• Palm trees in the Seychelles grow coconuts weighing over forty pounds.

• A Danish linguist, Rasmus Rask, compiled dictionaries in 28 of the 235 different languages he could speak.

• The world's first oil rig struck oil at Titusville, Pennsylvania, on August 28, 1859. On the same day in 1922 the United States scored another world first when station WEAF in New York City broadcast the world's first-ever radio commercial.

August 29

TONIGHT'S CURE

Spend spend spend. Tonight add up in your head, to the last cent, exactly how much money you spent last week. Remember every little item you bought and add it on as you go along, no matter how big or small the bill was. If you know how much cash you had at the start of the week and how much you have left at the end you should be able to account for all your expenses. Don't worry, because you won't! But the sheer effort will send you to sleep and you never know, you may have stopped worrying about where the money's all gone.

TONIGHT'S TRIVIA

• One morning, in 1943, a temperature change of over eighty degrees took place within two minutes in South Dakota.

• In the Middle Ages nearly one day in three was a holiday.

• During the dissection of a toad almost four hundred ants were found in its stomach.

• Water jets used in the manufacture of high-carbon steel are strong enough to blast a hole in a wooden plank.

August 30

TONIGHT'S CURE

Copy book. Copying is one of the most exacting and tedious occupations and as such it makes an ideal cure for insomnia. Take a piece of paper, a pencil, and a book with you to bed tonight. Choose any page from the book at random and set to work copying down, word for word, exactly what is on that page. Press on until you have copied at least one page. Put out the light and attempt to go to sleep. If you are still awake after half an hour, then turn on the light and copy another page.

TONIGHT'S TRIVIA

• If you wished to break off an engagement in medieval times, you sent a sprig of lilac to your betrothed.
• Bears have been known to climb telegraph poles after mistaking the buzzing of the wires for that of bees.
• Nero took part in the Olympic Games, that is he won a first prize, although he never actually ran one race.
• Excluding the United States, India is the leading film producing country in the world.

August 31

TONIGHT'S CURE

Temperature change. Medical evidence proves that at night your body drops in temperature when it is ready to go to bed. So tonight take your temperature throughout the evening and note the point when it actually drops. This is your body's way of telling you it is time for bed and you shouldn't have any trouble getting to sleep.

TONIGHT'S TRIVIA

• A piglet weighs three pounds at birth and two hundred pounds at six months.
• A book published in 1916 about the state of Georgia was bound in the shape of that state's boundaries.
• In Switzerland the surname of William Tell means mad.
• If the root system of a pumpkin plant were stretched out it would be almost twelve miles long.

September 1

TONIGHT'S CURE

Protein food. If you have the unfortunate habit of waking up in the middle of the night and are unable to fall asleep again, keep some protein food beside your bed to eat when you awake. Yogurt is ideal, especially natural yogurt, for it is said to have special properties that purify the blood. Cheese is another valuable protein food, and peanuts are rich in protein too. You may wish to have some milk as well to wash down your solid food, but avoid anything that contains sugar as this will give you energy and keep you awake.

TONIGHT'S TRIVIA

• The practice of branding criminals with a hot iron was not abolished in China until 1905.

• Christian Heinrich, of Lubeck, Germany, was able to talk when he was eight weeks old, and he could recite passages from the Bible by his first birthday.

• A chaffinch nest, built entirely of confetti, was discovered in 1940.

• Buying an automobile today costs more than it cost to equip Columbus's first voyage to the New World.

September 2

. . . .

TONIGHT'S CURE

Negative. When your head is buzzing with so many ideas that you can't sleep just close your eyes and let your mind go completely blank. Then think only in terms of grey, so everything you see looks rather like a negative that has been overexposed. Breathe very deeply and regularly and prevent the greyness from taking on any exact or familiar shape. As soon as it does, think back to blank again, remembering to breathe deeply all the time.

TONIGHT'S TRIVIA

• Pyritology is the name given to a study of blow pipes.

• The Colossus of Rhodes, one of the seven ancient wonders of the world, was stolen by invaders and melted down.

• Grasshoppers have white blood.

• It has been estimated that the receipts from illegal gambling in the United States is greater than the combined revenue of the top seventy-five industrial organizations in the country.

September 3

TONIGHT'S CURE

Heavy breathing. No, this has nothing to do with late night phone calls; it's a cure aimed at helping you get to sleep tonight. Lie on your back, close your eyes, open your mouth, and relax. Now breathe in very slowly through your mouth and count to ten. Hold your breath for five, then breathe out through your nose to a count of ten. Now breathe in through your nose and out through your mouth. Then in through the mouth and out through the nose. Keep to this routine of nose, mouth, mouth, nose, nose, mouth, and keep counting while you breathe.

TONIGHT'S TRIVIA

• Black and yellow have a stronger visual impact than black and white.
• Gasoline will extinguish a fire in a bale of cotton more efficiently than would water.
• Half the wealth of the world is held by just four countries that together have less than 15 percent of the entire human population.
• An average of nine inches more snow falls in Santa Fe, New Mexico, each year than falls in New Haven, Connecticut.

September 4

TONIGHT'S CURE

Accounts. One of the quickest methods of falling asleep is to do your accounts in bed. Nothing is better or faster at making you feel sleepy. If, however, this cure does not work for you, there is at least the compensation that your accounts will be completed and you'll have extra time during the day to do something much more exciting.

TONIGHT'S TRIVIA

• Yap islanders make sails for their boats by interlacing leaves of the pandanus tree.
• In the French Revolution a midget disguised as a baby acted as a spy and was carried through "enemy lines" undetected.
• To make one kilo of saffron you need 140,000 crocuses.
• Before corks were used, bottles were sealed by pouring oil into their necks.

September 5

TONIGHT'S CURE

Heartfelt. Tonight choose a famous classical play, perhaps one of Shakespeare's. Choose a particular speech that you like and set out to learn it by heart. Read the first line and say it over to yourself a couple of times. Read the next sentence and repeat that a couple of times. Now repeat the two sentences together. Read the third sentence. Repeat it a couple of times. Then repeat all three sentences without looking at the book. Continue like this until you have learned the whole speech. To test whether or not you know it well, turn out the light and recite the whole speech to yourself. Then repeat the speech every night to help you fall asleep.

TONIGHT'S TRIVIA

• The human body contains enough fat to make seven bars of soap.
• St. John the Evangelist was the only apostle to die a natural death.
• During the reign of George III, in England, sixty-five hundred tons of hair powder were used annually by the British Army.
• A common method of suicide in China used to be eating a pound of salt.

September 6

TONIGHT'S CURE

Mantras. If you are able to obtain a book on yoga you will find that it contains many mantras to help you sleep. One of these requires you to focus your attention between your eyes (with a piece of scotch tape stuck on your forehead as noted in a previous cure if it makes it easier) and to chant "Om tat sat" over and over again. This means "Om that is good"—Om being the Supreme Spirit of Hinduism.

TONIGHT'S TRIVIA

• Skiers are sometimes afflicted with a complaint known as "gamekeeper's thumb."
• One ruler of Morocco, Ismail the Bloodthirsty, had 888 children.
• The longest fangs of any snake are two inches long and belong to the Gabon viper.
• The *Mayflower* set sail from Plymouth, England, on September 6, 1620, with a party of 103 pilgrims bound for religious freedom and the New World. The first great American sculptor, Horatio

Greenough, was born on this day in 1620 and William McKinley, the twenty-fifth U. S. president, was shot dead on September 6, 1901.

September 7

. . . .

TONIGHT'S CURE

Leo Tolstoy. How often have you said to yourself that you must make the effort to read one of the great Russian classic novels? How often have you put it off until another time? Well, why not start one tonight? Choose one of Leo Tolstoy's works such as *War and Peace* or *Anna Karenina,* two books with a colossal number of pages. Settle yourself comfortably in bed and then attempt to read as much of the book as you can tonight. Set yourself a certain number of chapters to read and however sleepy you feel continue reading until you have achieved your target. Then put the book down and don't open it until bedtime tomorrow night.

TONIGHT'S TRIVIA

- An Irish brogue is a type of shoe.
- Bakers used to be liable to heavy fines if they gave short measure and therefore always baked one extra loaf, hence a baker's dozen.
- The James Gang made its famous raid on the First National Bank in Northfield, Minnesota, on September 7, 1876, and was shot to pieces by the townspeople. Jesse and his brother Frank managed to escape, however, and exactly five years later to the day Jesse held up his final train at Blue Cut, Missouri.
- Every U.S. president has worn eyeglasses.

September 8

. . . .

TONIGHT'S CURE

Cocktails. This evening invite the most boring friends you have for drinks. Make sure they're people who will talk long into the night, but who will not involve you in any discussion or argument to stimulate your brain. Let them bore you to death, and let the combination of their trivial chitchat and the alcohol lull you into sleep.

TONIGHT'S TRIVIA

- Jim Glass, of California, built a bicycle bed that had wheels and which you could pedal lying down.
- In order to capture the cracking of a glass on film, a camera

needs to shoot at a millionth of a second.

- Hilaire Belloc wrote his own epitaph:

When I am dead I hope it may be said,
His sins were scarlet, but his books were read.

- On September 8, 1664, the Dutch town of New Amsterdam surrendered to the British and promptly had its name changed to New York.

September 9

TONIGHT'S CURE

Anniversary. Tonight try to remember exactly what you were doing one year ago today. Look in your diary to see which day of the week it was. It might be your birthday, or an anniversary, so it may stand out in your mind, or it could be just an ordinary day on which nothing outstanding happened and about which you can remember nothing. If that's the case, cast your mind back over the past year and remember all the key events that have happened to you and your family. Why not note them down and then compare them with next year's list?

TONIGHT'S TRIVIA

- The Greeks had a tradition according to which newly married couples shared a quince at their wedding feast.
- Israel is the only country in the world to have compulsory military service for women.
- California, the state with the highest human population and the largest population of chickens in the United States, achieved its statehood on September 9, 1850.
- In 1610 there were only 350 people living in the American colonies.

September 10

TONIGHT'S CURE

Funny ha ha. Tonight you get your chance to be the leading celebrity on a TV talk show. You've got to fill the show with all the hilarious side-splitting things that have ever happened to you. OK, what do you choose? Where do you begin? Lie back on your pillow and just think of every amusing incident and scrape you've been in. They may not have been much of a laugh at the time, but they sure seem funny now. Weave them into an entertaining narrative and maybe try it out on your friends next time you have a get-together. Who knows, you could end up a star.

TONIGHT'S TRIVIA

- The peacock has been a symbol of resurrection for centuries.
- Young Spartan men were made to line up naked every month to see if they were overweight.
- In 1964 an aircraft flying over Chicago was struck by lightning five times in a space of twenty minutes without any damage being caused.
- The first head of the U.S. Post Office was Benjamin Franklin.

September 11

TONIGHT'S CURE

M T. As you lie in the dark, listen to the ticking of your clock. Count each of the ticks and then suddenly stop counting, but continue listening. Switch your thoughts to something totally unconnected and then let your mind go completely blank. Now start to focus your mind on the two letters *M* and *T.* Try to see them with your mind's eye. Say them to yourself over and over again, picking up the rhythm of the clock once more, saying *M T, M T, M T, M T.* This will gradually become *empty, empty,* and you'll find that your mind too will become empty as you drift into a deep sleep.

TONIGHT'S TRIVIA

- Cats cannot taste sweet food.
- The common spider has six hundred silk glands and can lay six hundred eggs at one time.
- The hurricane plant has holes in its leaves that prevent it from being damaged in any wind.
- September 11, 1928, saw the world's first television play. Station WGY in Schenectady, New York, broadcast *The Queen's Messenger,* a two-character play with four actors. (The two extra actors were needed for the close-up shots of the characters' hands since the cameras could not move.)

September 12

TONIGHT'S CURE

Asana. *Asana* is the Indian word for posture, and there are many postures you can adopt which will help you sleep. One of these is called· *The Cobra.* When you are ready for bed, lie face downward on the floor, with your forehead touching the floor. Then slowly raise your head and neck and tilt your head back. Place the palms of your hands flat on the floor directly under your shoulders to support you and keep tilting your head back as if you were trying to see your feet. Arch your back as far as it will go without stretching or straining, pushing down on your palms as you do so, until your arms are straight. Throughout the exercize your legs remain flat on the floor. When you've completed the exercise, gently relax, lowering yourself down into your original position. Now rest for one minute and then repeat.

TONIGHT'S TRIVIA

• The oldest moon rock brought back to earth was found to contain twenty times more uranium and potassium than any other moon rock previously studied.
• Dachshunds were kept by Egyptians four thousand years ago.
• Cow's milk contains twice as much protein as human milk.
• Research shows that men are twice as likely to fall out of hospital beds as women.

September 13

TONIGHT'S CURE

Day by day. As you lie in bed tonight, calculate how many days you have actually been alive. This is not as hard as it may sound. Simply multiply the number of years that you have been alive by 365 and you will get a rough estimate of how many days you have lived. Now multiply this figure by twenty-four to get the number of hours, multiply that figure by sixty to get the number of minutes, multiply that total by sixty again and you get the number of seconds. All this must be done in your head, in the dark, although you may use your fingers if they're of any help with numbers of this size!

TONIGHT'S TRIVIA

• In the Dominican Republic it takes one day to obtain a divorce.
• Male seals are called bulls and the females are called cows, but their young are called pups.
• Dogs wag their tails when they are pleased, cats when they are angry.
• A newly hatched crocodile is three times larger than its egg.

September 14

TONIGHT'S CURE

Empty glass. Have you ever wondered what it would be like to be transparent and to be able to see everything that goes on inside your body? Well tonight try to imagine that your body is made of glass and that the air you breathe in is very cloudy. Breath in a cloud of air that will waft gently into your body and continue inhaling so your body becomes completely filled with this cloudy vapor. Remember, it must get right down to your feet and toes and you have to fill your body right to the top of your head. Concentrate on breathing deeply and circulate this air throughout your body into every extremity and recess.

TONIGHT'S TRIVIA

• One bucket of water could produce enough fog to cover 104 square miles.

• Any five-digit number multiplied by 11 and then multiplied again by 9,091 will reappear twice in the product.

• In 1060 a coin was minted in England in the shape of a four-leaf clover so that each "leaf" could be broken off and used separately.

• Caterpillars have over two thousand muscles.

September 15

TONIGHT'S CURE

Olive oil. Olive oil is a well-known remedy for insomnia; the prescribed dosage is one spoonful after your evening meal and another one before going to bed. However, if like me you cannot stomach this, then you can take the two spoonfuls in a more palatable way. Don't bother to separate the two doses, just mix the two spoonfuls with a dessertspoon of cocoa powder or malted milk powder to make a paste, then mix this with boiled milk and drink it about one hour before going to bed.

TONIGHT'S TRIVIA

• Ten-thousand-year-old seeds have been successfully grown in laboratories.

• Denim material was originally made in Nimes, France, and originally called *De Nimes*.

• In 1888 the Sultan of Turkey became the first royal motorist.

• Packaged frozen foods were invented by Clarence Birdseye.

September 16

TONIGHT'S CURE

Limb by limb. If it's tension in your arms and legs that's keeping you awake, stretch, lift, and wiggle each limb in turn, and then let it relax. Start with the toes on your left foot, then move up your left side and down your right side ending with your right foot. Stretch each limb as far as it will go and then let it completely relax before you move on to the next one.

TONIGHT'S TRIVIA

• In July, 1979, an American hen laid an egg which contained nine yolks.

• The right side of your brain controls the left side of your body and vice-versa.

• Christianity has a larger number of followers than any other religion.

• The first novel ever written on a typewriter was *The Adventures of Tom Sawyer,* which Mark Twain typed by himself on a Remington machine in 1875.

September 17

TONIGHT'S CURE

Alphabetical wardrobe. After you've undressed and gotten into bed tonight, spare a thought for your clothes. Check first that your wardrobe door is firmly closed and then turn out your light. Starting a list in alphabetical order, take an item of clothing or footwear for every letter of the alphabet, starting with *A* for ankle sock, *B* for briefs, *C* for corset, and so on. Then say the complete list in reverse order when you have reached the end.

TONIGHT'S TRIVIA

• The Marquis de Pelier spent fifty years in prison for whistling at Queen Marie Antoinette.

• An egg will float in a glass of water to which sugar has been added.

• The coastline of Canada is six times longer than the coastline of the world's smallest continent, Australia.

• The third hand of a watch is the second hand.

September 18

TONIGHT'S CURE

Primrose tea. For anyone who is very high strung or susceptible to nervous tension, primrose tea is an excellent remedy to help you rest. It is available in any drugstore and is not addictive. Lime blossom tea is another harmless, pleasant drink, and is particularly effective if a tiny pinch of skullcap is added. These natural herbs have been used with great success for centuries. If modern cures aren't helping you, give these old-world brews a try!

TONIGHT'S TRIVIA

• Hurricanes can be fifty times stronger than all other winds blowing at one time put together.
• Aspirin occurs naturally on the barks of certain trees.
• When the great Palace of Versailles was built it had no bathrooms or lavatories.
• Of all the species of shark in the seas less than ten have jaws capable of eating a man, and even less have the desire.

September 19

TONIGHT'S CURE

Gray's elegy. One of the great literary remedies for insomnia is to read the poem by the English poet Thomas Gray, entitled *Elegy Written in a Country Churchyard*. It has thirty-two verses but many people are unable to get beyond the first line. However, if you are able to learn the poem, or if you know it already, try repeating it in the alphabetical progression of the initial letter of each line, so that the first stanza will thus read:
Along the heath and near his fav'rite tree,
And all that beauty, all that wealth e'er gave,
And all the air a solemn stillness holds,
And drowsy tinklings lull the distant folds.

TONIGHT'S TRIVIA

• The Hundred Years War lasted 114 years.
• Over forty-two million people died during the Black Death in the thirteenth century.
• The Golden Gate Bridge in San Francisco averages one suicide per month.
• Hero Zzyzzx is the last name in the Madison, Wisconsin,

telephone directory. It's his real name, and is an amalgam of Finnish, Lithuanian, Russian, French, and German.

September 20

TONIGHT'S CURE

Carole's husband. Read this problem tonight, when you're in bed, then turn out the light and try to solve it.

Carole is twenty-four years old. She is twice as old as Clarence was when she was as old as he is now. How old is Clarence?*

TONIGHT'S TRIVIA

- In 1884 there was an earthquake in Great Britain that killed four people.
- If you touch the leaves of the sensitive plant they move away from you.
- In Siberia solid blocks of tea were once used as currency.
- American Indians live on their land tax free.

*Solution: Clarence is eighteen.

September 21

TONIGHT'S CURE

Canoeing. One of the most frequent nightmares is the one in which we are trying desperately to escape some unseen menace while remaining rooted to the spot. When we wake up from this nightmare we usually feel exhausted, so in this cure the idea is to exhaust yourself mentally *before* you go to sleep. Start by imagining you are in a canoe battling against a river with a very strong current. Breathe in and out very deeply as you paddle the canoe. Imagine that the paddling is difficult because of the force of the current. Take one stroke with each breath, heaving as hard as you can. You have to continue paddling until you reach the campsite, which is in view, but it's hard going and you're getting more tired with each stroke.

TONIGHT'S TRIVIA

- Chemically, the closest substance to human blood is seawater.
- The tenth U.S. president, John Tyler, had fifteen children.
- Spaniards used to clean their teeth with urine.
- Nearly every Moslem family has at least one child named Muhammad.

September 22

TONIGHT'S CURE

Chatter. Tonight is a perfect night for reliving a conversation that you've recently had with a friend. First picture the situation in your mind's eye. What were you both wearing? Where did the conversation take place? What did you start talking about? When the conversation is rolling, let it wander off onto another track and imagine how you could conduct this new conversation. Then gradually drop out of it yourself and let your friend completely monopolize what is being said.

TONIGHT'S TRIVIA

• Many natives in central Africa carve chairs out of solid blocks of wood.
• In British Columbia you can be sentenced to two hours in the stocks for buying an ice cream or a bag of peanuts.
• The income-tax rate in the Gulf state of Bahrain is nil.
• Five tons of ore-bearing rock will yield one piece of gold the size of a small button.

September 23

TONIGHT'S CURE

Pollen cakes. Pollen cakes are eaten at night by the Burmese in the belief that these cakes induce sleep. A great deal of research has been undertaken recently regarding the effects of pollen. Pollen cakes were first made by the Chinese. To make a pollen cake spread a thick layer of honey onto a flat surface, then alternate layers of pollen and honey until you have six layers in thickness. Then knead this like a dough, until it ends up rather like a pancake. The substance should be left to dry for five days and then cut up into strips to be eaten whenever health or insomnia demand.

TONIGHT'S TRIVIA

• Chickens are the only animals you eat both before they are born and after they are dead.
• The practice of castrating choristers was only stopped a century ago.
• The great English writer, Charles Dickens, would only write facing northward.
• Heroin was originally thought to be a cure for opium addiction.

September 24

TONIGHT'S CURE

Revolving. Take a trip to the amusement park tonight without leaving your bed. All you have to do is lie on your side with your knees bent and your hands placed lightly and loosely in front of your chest. Now close your eyes and imagine that the bed is a car that turns on a turntable and that it is slowly rotating to the left. Feel yourself moving round and round, gradually gaining speed. It is a very easy feeling to achieve. You may find yourself spinning to the right, but most people naturally feel as if they are spinning counterclockwise. Just lie there and let the movement send you off to sleep.

TONIGHT'S TRIVIA

• In the New Testament the only miracle referred to by all four evangelists is the feeding of the five thousand.
• In the first juvenile court the first case heard was that of a youngster accused of shouting "Celery!" in the street.
• In Britain, during the Middle Ages, it was illegal to store French and Spanish wine in the same cellar.
• Bedouin Arabs made conflicting witnesses lick a red-hot bar of iron.

September 25

TONIGHT'S CURE

Dame Nikki Elsom's remedy. This cure was invented by the great British eccentric and wit, the outrageous Dame Nikki Elsom from northern England. However, this is not to be recommended for anyone with a nervous disposition. Dame Nikki's cure is to take each part of your anatomy in turn and name any medical operation that could be performed on that part of your body. Start with a "full-frontal lobotomy" and continue until removal of an ingrown toenail. Very few people get past "hysterectomy."

TONIGHT'S TRIVIA

• The average man has thirty-two teeth.
• Ten times as many men as women are color-blind.·
• Seals only fall asleep for intervals of one and one-half minutes.
• President Carter saw a UFO in 1969 during his birth month.

September 26

TONIGHT'S CURE

Elbow and shoulder meet. Does the top part of your body need a workout before you settle down to sleep? If you think that might help, here's a simple routine you can do in bed.

First of all, sit up and lay your head as far back as it will go, giving your neck a really good stretch. Then rotate your shoulders in a circular motion, first forward and then back. Don't worry if the bones crack slightly, they're just loosening up. Now put your shoulders back as far as they will go, with your elbows behind you, and try to make them touch. Repeat this routine three or four times and then see how you sleep.

TONIGHT'S TRIVIA

• Marcel Proust only wrote in bed, in a soundproof bedroom.
• There are enough stones in the Great Pyramid at Cheops to build a wall, three feet high, all round the frontiers of France.
• The motor giant, Henry Ford, once tried to buy the Eiffel Tower and ship it to America.
• Emeralds were once thought to facilitate childbirth if they were worn by the expectant mother.

September 27

TONIGHT'S CURE

One million. Are you the sort of person whose mind boggles when you're confronted with huge numbers? If you are then this cure's for you. Start counting at nine-hundred and ninety-five thousand one-hundred and one, and count in ones until you reach the number one million. Do not, however, become lazy and abbreviate the number to ease counting. You have to say: "nine-hundred and ninety-five thousand one-hundred and one" and so on, and if you lose count, you must return to your starting point.

TONIGHT'S TRIVIA

• The horse was native to America, but it died out there about ten thousand years ago and had to be reintroduced in the sixteenth century.
• The word *and* occurs in the Bible 46,227 times.
• The Babylonian zero was written like our colon (:).
• There are over four thousand items of assorted space instruments and debris littering outer space.

September 28

TONIGHT'S CURE

Cycle. Riding a bicycle is an excellent and enjoyable method of using up energy. Today forget about automobiles, cabs, and any other kind of transportation except the bicycle. Cycle to work, cycle to the shops, and cycle to visit friends. At night before going to bed, or earlier in the evening, go for a long cycle ride, preferably somewhere with a calm, peaceful view, which will help you unwind.

TONIGHT'S TRIVIA

• In Germany there is a breed of flea that lives only in beer mats.
• General Dwight Eisenhower had the five stars of his rank on the collar of his pajamas.
• If you chew gum while peeling onions it will prevent you from crying.
• If you put a drop of whisky on the back of a scorpion it will sting itself to death.

September 29

TONIGHT'S CURE

Quick march. Marching might seem a dumb way of getting to sleep, but the exercise and the rhythm will help you unwind before you settle down. Before getting into bed, stand by the side of your bed and start to march slowly. Lift your legs as high as you can so your knees come up to your chest. Count each left and right step as your feet touch the ground and count up to five hundred before you stop and get into bed.

TONIGHT'S TRIVIA

• Our sun is thirty thousand light-years away from the center of the Milky Way.
• Our nearest neighboring star is 25 million miles away.
• Our modern telescopes allow us to look at galaxies 4 billion light years away.
• The movies' first singing cowboy, Gene Autry, was born on September 29, 1907, and another U.S. singer, Jerry Lee Lewis, was born in Ferriday, Louisiana, on this date in 1935.

September 30

TONIGHT'S CURE

Rowing. The lazy, rhythmical swing of rowing a boat on a warm afternoon can help send you to sleep at night. All you have to do is to sit up in the dark and clasp your hands under your knees. Now just start to swing your body backwards and forwards in a steady, comfortable rhythm. Finally close your eyes and imagine yourself rowing on a beautiful summer afternoon, and just row yourself to sleep like this.

TONIGHT'S TRIVIA

• On September 30, 1961, the Mayor of Jackson County, Oregon, sent a check for $1.96 to a London trading company. The sum represented Jackson County's share of the bill for the tea emptied into Boston harbor during the Boston Tea Party 188 years earlier.
• Poltergeists frequently manifest their presence through the abnormal behavior of young girls.
• The Library of Congress contains 73 million items, housed on 350 miles of shelving.
• The odds against a mother producing quadruplets are one in six-hundred thousand.

October 1

TONIGHT'S CURE

Speaking clock. Before turning out your light tonight look at your watch and note the exact time. Now turn out the light, lie down in a comfortable position, and imagine that you are the speaking clock. Say "At the third stroke it will be eleven twenty-six and ten seconds, beep, beep, beep. At the third stroke it will be eleven twenty-six and twenty seconds, beep, beep, beep. At the third stroke it will be eleven twenty-six and thirty seconds, beep, beep, beep." Count like this for as long as you can. Very few people get past five minutes before they are asleep.

TONIGHT'S TRIVIA

• Doris Day began her career as a dancer after she had been in the hospital with a broken leg.
• Rubber is used in the manufacture of chewing gum.

- One tenth century ruler of China had four pupils, two in each eye.
- Whale meat is very rich in vitamin C.

October 2

TONIGHT'S CURE

Lavender. The smell of lavender has well-known soporific qualities. So place a few bunches of fresh lavender in vases of water around your room tonight. Alternatively put some small muslin bags of dried lavender under your pillow. Then when you lie down to go to sleep let the fragrance fill your mind and relax your body. Dream of fragrant fields filled with lavender.

TONIGHT'S TRIVIA

- Sea otters have two fur coats.
- Theodore Roosevelt was Eleanor Roosevelt's uncle.
- Only a century after Muhammad's death one-third of the world had been converted to Islam.
- Gunpowder was first used during battle in 1346.

October 3

TONIGHT'S CURE

Dream return. All of us have a dream every night, even if we do not remember it in the morning. Sometimes we remember a dream very vividly but do not know why. Often a dream can be very enjoyable and we get quite annoyed when we are woken up and have to leave the events. It is, however, quite easy to return to a dream. So if you have had a pleasant dream recently, close your eyes when you settle down tonight and think about what happened, trying to get back into the story where you left off.

TONIGHT'S TRIVIA

- The oldest international cricket match in the world was played between the United States and Canada in 1844.
- Some bamboos in southeast Asia can grow over a yard a day.
- The longest recorded stroke of lightning ran for twenty miles across the sky.
- Crows can distinguish a man with a gun from a man without one.

October 4

TONIGHT'S CURE

Foot massage. Foot massage is an excellent method of relaxing your tired and aching muscles at night. If you want to try this first lift your right foot onto your left knee. Now massage the sole of your foot using the knuckles of your right hand, pressing very hard. This may feel uncomfortable, but it will be relieving tension in your foot. Next, grasp each of the toes and move them up and down and side to side, running your fingers in between each toe. Now massage the top of your foot with your finger tips, using a circular motion moving in one direction. Next push your fingertips right into the sole of your foot and massage this area. Finally massage your ankle, moving your foot in a circular motion as you do so. Then repeat this with your other foot.

TONIGHT'S TRIVIA

• Three-quarters of the world's plants grow under the sea.
• It is impossible for human skin to be completely black.
• X rays were discovered accidentally when a physicist's wife put her hand in the way.
• There were several eunuchs who have led perfectly normal sex lives.

October 5

TONIGHT'S CURE

Aura. Have you ever wondered what it would be like to be surrounded by a protective aura that cocooned you completely from the outside world? If you haven't, then try imagining this tonight. Your aura shelters you completely from all the harms of the world outside. It is impervious to the elements, to violence of any sort, and it also renders you invisible. So, step inside this aura and feel its warmth and strength. Then transport yourself to any destination you choose to explore and examine the most dangerous places imaginable with no fear of harm.

TONIGHT'S TRIVIA

• Natives of New Guinea smoke their cigarettes from the side.
• In Montoire, France, there is a speaking well that, when spoken into, will repeat whole phrases.
• Until 1790 only three students at a time were admitted to the Harvard University library.

• The largest inhabited castle in the world is Windsor Castle, in England, one of the homes of Queen Elizabeth II.

October 6

. . . .

TONIGHT'S CURE

Omelet. Have a light meal tonight and. then try this cure before you go to bed. Half an hour before bedtime make yourself an omelet with at least two eggs and a little milk. Cook it with a little oil and eat it as soon as it's ready, with one slice of bread. Wash it down with milk and water, but not with anything stimulating like tea or coffee. Then let yourself unwind while you digest this before retiring to bed.

TONIGHT'S TRIVIA

• Sodium burns in water but not in paraffin.
• The first recorded murder trial took place in 1700 B.C.
• One Roman cure for epilepsy was to drink fresh gladiator's blood.
• Bowling was once forbidden on Sundays.

October 7

. . . .

TONIGHT'S CURE

Palindromes. For those whose level of mental activity prevents them from falling asleep, here's a cure that should fully occupy all their intellectual powers, and rapidly send them to sleep—palindromes. A palindrome is a word that is spelled the same backward and forward. The longest palindrome in our language is *redivider* and the most famous sentences are *Madam, I'm Adam*, and *Able was I ere I saw Elba*. See how many palindromes you can make. Think of palindromic names to start with, but see if you can create a whole palindrome sentence before you fall asleep.

TONIGHT'S TRIVIA

• Most of the automobile trips made. in the United States are for journeys of less than five miles.
• Hawaiian flower necklaces often contain as many as five hundred flowers.
• There are twenty-six countries in the world with no coastline.
• The first astronauts in Skylab carried travel sickness pills.

October 8

TONIGHT'S CURE

Who's who? Read this puzzle, then turn out the light and solve it.

Two people get into bed together. One is the father of the other person's son. How are these two people related?

TONIGHT'S TRIVIA

• An employee at the Louvre once stole the *Mona Lisa* and tried to sell it for $100,000.

• Snails only mate once in a lifetime, but the act can take twelve hours.

• Polar bears can swim faster than the speed achieved by an Olympic swimmer.

• Wire wool burns faster than sheep's wool.

*Solution: They are husband and wife.

October 9

TONIGHT'S CURE

Candlelight. Candlelight has a very soothing, soporific effect, as other cures have shown. So place a lighted candle beside your bed tonight and turn out every other source of light. Choose a book that has relatively small print and attempt to read it by the light of the candle. Before long you will feel incredibly tired and may only have time to blow out the candle before you drift off to sle....

TONIGHT'S TRIVIA

• Shakespeare's daughter could not read.

• Dandelions are rich in vitamin A.

• Eau de Cologne was originally developed as protection against the plague.

• Cooked brussel sprouts have lost 90 percent of their original vitamin content.

October 10

TONIGHT'S CURE

Love. One of the greatest gifts that you can wish for anybody is not great fortune, but the pleasure of love. The experience of loving and being loved in return is a feeling which we hopefully all enjoy at some time in our lives, and no matter how fleeting it may be, the sensation is blissful just the same. Tonight then, visualize a very personal relationship which involved a person for whom you have felt a great love. Relive the joys and pleasure of that time of great happiness in your life, and if that person happens to be beside you now, reach out and hold his or her hand.

TONIGHT'S TRIVIA

• Many anthropologists believe that early man could sing before he could speak.

• Most UFOs are spotted at times when Mars is nearest the earth.

• Psychological study shows that women talk about men three times more often than men talk about women.

• On October 10, 1961, a ninety-foot high volcano suddenly appeared on Tristan da Cunha Island in the Atlantic.

October 11

TONIGHT'S CURE

Way to the stars. If it's a clear night tonight try to find your way to sleep by traveling the way to the stars. Lie on your back and look up at the night sky. Gaze up at the stars and try to appreciate how far away they are. The sun is 90 million miles away and the nearest stars are even further than that. This distance is totally incomprehensible to most of us and impossible to imagine. However, let this thought virtually fill your mind. Say to yourself: "If I should fall I would go up and up and up." Concentrate on this one idea until you feel the stars drawing you toward them. Feel yourself being pulled as the earth slips away from you as you drift into the heavens and space engulfs you completely.

TONIGHT'S TRIVIA

• The longest place name in New Zealand is *Tuamatawhakatangihangakoauauotamateapokaiwhenuakitanatahu*.

• A snail can crawl over a razor blade without cutting itself.

• Gold is indestructible—the mask of Agamemnon was found after three thousand years in perfect condition.

• On October 11, 1884, H. J. Heinz, of beans fame, came into the world. Forty years later Eleanor Roosevelt was born, while on the same date in 1973 two dock workers in Pascaquola, Mississippi, were kidnapped by a UFO and examined by its occupants for twenty minutes before being returned to earth.

October 12

TONIGHT'S CURE

Telepathy. This cure can be undertaken with a sleeping partner until you both feel tired. Both lie on your back with the light out, or you can lie facing each other if it makes it easier. Both think of a word. Both think hard for one minute. After this time both count in unison—five, four, three, two, one—and shout out the word you had in your mind. Is it the same? If not, don't worry, just do it again. Then both think of a number, an animal, a state, a president, a friend, a food, etc.

TONIGHT'S TRIVIA

• John Massis of Belgium could pull a thirty-six-ton train with his teeth.
• There are an estimated total of 28 million cats in America.
• Before myxomatosis in 1951, there were 100 billion rabbits in Australia.
• Robert E. Lee died on October 12, 1870, the day on which the New World had been "discovered" by Christopher Columbus in 1492.

October 13

TONIGHT'S CURE

Salad days. You probably know how refreshing the juice of certain fruits and vegetables feels on your skin when you are eating them, and these can have the same soothing effect at night when you want to go to sleep.

Take half a lemon to bed with you tonight and without squeezing it, rub it lightly over your face. Then take a chunk of cucumber and rub that lightly over your face as well. You will find them both very cool and soothing. Now take two slices of cucumber and place one on each eyelid. Lie on your back with your eyes closed and feel the coolness of the cucumber being absorbed into your body. After ten to fifteen minutes remove the slices and see if you can fall asleep.

TONIGHT'S TRIVIA

• In France a black eye is called a poached eye.
• The ancient Chinese believed that sperm came from the brain.
• In early Europe potatoes were blamed for giving the eater syphilis.

- Bombay duck is made from fried fish.

October 14

TONIGHT'S CURE

Psychic journey. You may have heard about people who claim to project themselves in their sleep, and though you can't hope to match them instantly, try to summon your powers of concentration to help you. Think of a friend or a local place that you wish to visit. Lie comfortably in a warm bed and say to yourself, "I am getting out of bed...I am walking across the room...I am opening the door...I am going downstairs...I am opening the front door...I am walking down the street..." Do this throughout the complete journey until you reach your destination. If this has worked you will see, in your mind, exactly what your friend is doing. If this cure hasn't had quite this effect, it will still have taken your mind off your other worries and anxieties enough to let you get to sleep more easily.

TONIGHT'S TRIVIA

- Koala bears get their name from the aborigine term for no drink.
- The first man to fly faster than the speed of sound hurtled through the air over Edwards Air Force Base in California on October 14,1947, when pilot Chuck Yeager flew at 670 miles per hour or Mach 1.015.
- The United States had no national anthem until 1931.
- In 1648 actors who performed in public could be flogged.

October 15

TONIGHT'S CURE

Interview. You may have already tried imagining you are a celebrity on a talk show, but tonight's your chance to host a late-night talk show. You have to decide which celebrity you want to interview. Is it a top movie star, or maybe an Olympic champion? No matter who it is, you have to work out exactly what questions you're going to ask. Try to imagine yourself in the studio waiting for the cue to indicate that you're on the air. How would you make your guest feel at east? What are your first words to your TV audience? OK ten seconds to go...five...and on you go.

TONIGHT'S TRIVIA

- Deimos, one of the moons of Mars, sets and rises twice daily.

- Horses show they are angry by putting their ears back.
- In 1971 a primitive tribe was discovered in the Philippines that did not farm, had no animals, lived without clothes, and had never seen a wheel.
- An unfortunate Miss Fanny Miles of Cincinnati, Ohio, had feet which were over two feet long.

October 16

TONIGHT'S CURE

Yawning. When we yawn it is usually a sign that we are tired and need some sleep. You may not be yawning now, but you can *make* yourself yawn very easily. Try it and you'll find that once you start yawning, it will be impossible to stop. The more you yawn, the more tired you will feel, and this will make you fall asleep in no time.

TONIGHT'S TRIVIA

- Scientists say that a Chihuahua is a rodent, not a dog.
- A starfish can turn its stomach inside out.
- Literally one person in a million has an IQ of 180.
- One of the rules of the club established by the ancient scientist Pythagoras was that no member was allowed to poke a fire with an object made of iron.

October 17

TONIGHT'S CURE

Pillow speaker. Learning while you sleep has been in practice for some time and this cure uses the same principle—pillow speakers. These are now widely available, fairly inexpensive, and are particularly effective if you have a tape of a story being read to you, or even a sleep cassette which will hypnotize you into slumber. With a pillow speaker you can listen to a tape as you doze off—but the narrator will continue to impart information directly into your subconscious mind all through the night—so you could wake up brainier in the morning after a good night's sleep.

TONIGHT'S TRIVIA

- Beethoven used to stimulate his brain with ice.
- The nail on your middle finger grows faster than any other nail on your hands or feet.

- Fifteen buildings were hit by meteorites during the last century.
- In western Africa the Matani tribe used to play football with a skull.

October 18

TONIGHT'S CURE

Bird's nest. There's something so warm and welcoming about even the tiniest bird's nest. The fledglings seem so secure and safe with their parents guarding and feeding them. Imagine you are a tiny bird, warm and snug in your nest. Imagine you are covered in feathers and are snuggled up close to the other birds around you. Try to visualize how big everything else appears to your bird's-eye view. Picture the trees, the leaves, and everything else around you. Imagine the sense of freedom at being able to fly for the first time and try to capture the thrill of the lightness of your body that enables you to glide through the air. Launch yourself into the air for a breathtaking flight and then return to the warmth and comfort of your own cozy nest.

TONIGHT'S TRIVIA

- If all the gold that has ever been mined was totaled together it would only be equal to the amount of metal produced by the American steel industry in two hours.
- There is no word in our language that rhymes with the word *oblige*.
- Compared with the rise in the cost of living coffee is still the same price as it was three hundred years ago.
- Henry Matisse's idiosyncratic painting *Le Bateau* went on display in the Museum of Modern Art in New York on October 18, 1961. However, it was only forty-six days and 116,000 visitors later that it was realized that the work had been displayed upside down!

October 19

TONIGHT'S CURE

Reverse sdrow. Have fun with words tonight while you're lying awake in bed. Say your own name backwards and see how different it sounds, like mine which is Luap Semaj. Play with your new name on your tongue. It may even sound amusing, for example, if your name is Gordon Gibb, it will turn into Nodrog Bbig. Now reverse the names of all the members of your family to see how strange they sound. Then attempt to say entire sentences in reverse, ti si ton oot tluciffid.

TONIGHT'S TRIVIA

• Monkeys are the only animals to have color vision equal to that of man.

• The nerve endings in the brain are equivalent to a telephone exchange connected to every person in the world.

• Blood is over 90 percent water.

• The United States finally won her independence on October 19, 1781, when the British Army, under Lord Cornwallis, finally ran out of ammunition and surrendered. By a strange irony it was on exactly the same day in 1812 that Napoleon Bonaparte's army began its disastrous retreat from Moscow—both events marked the end of grandiose imperial dreams.

October 20

TONIGHT'S CURE

Stone yourself. Many of the cures deal with loosening and relaxing your body, but this one works in the opposite way. Your aim tonight is to try to turn yourself into stone. Lie on your back or side, whichever is more comfortable for you. (It is never advisable to sleep on your front as this restricts breathing and can be harmful to your neck muscles.) Breathe deeply and imagine that with each exhalation a part of your anatomy is turning to stone. Breathe in and breathe out. Your toes have turned to stone and feel very heavy. Breathe in, breathe out. Your feet have turned to stone. Breathe in, breathe out. Your ankles have turned to stone. Continue until your calves, knees, thighs, and every part of your body feels as if it has turned to stone. Finally let your eyes turn to stone. Let them become so heavy that it's impossible to keep them open and then fall asleep like a fallen statue.

TONIGHT'S TRIVIA

• A submarine cannot make radio contact with land while it is under water.

• A Boeing 747, sometimes called the Jumbo Jet, weighs the equivalent of seventy elephants.

• The polecat was originally called *poulechat* because it fed on poultry.

• The planet Uranus was not given a name until 1850.

October 21

TONIGHT'S CURE

Director cure. Tonight you have the chance to make the ultimate movie—the movie about *you*. Imagine that you are a top movie director in Hollywood, and are about to make a movie of your own life story. Make a mental list of all the key events that have happened in your life that you want to include, and more important, list all the people who have played a major role in your life story. Picture yourself holding auditions for the parts. Take each of your friends and relatives that are going to be in the story and decide which famous star you will cast to play each part. Katherine Hepburn as your mother, James Stewart as your father, Elizabeth Taylor as your sister, and so on. Then once you've cast the movie get to work on the script—tomorrow night perhaps?

TONIGHT'S TRIVIA

• Water contained in Australian artesian wells fell as rain over six thousand years ago.
• Homer is said to have died of shame after being unable to answer a riddle.
• Airplanes benefit from a dose of caster oil every now and then.
• Goldfish are able to remember things better in cold water than in warm water.

October 22

TONIGHT'S CURE

Mmmmmmmmmmmmmmmm. Once in bed tonight close your eyes and relax completely. Now start to hum very gently, holding any single note that comes most naturally to you. Feel it vibrate in your nose and the back of your throat. Take deep breaths and hum until your lungs are completely empty. Experiment with the vibrations but maintain your monatone note so that you are continually saying *mmmmmmmmmmmmmmmmmmmmmmmmm*. Raise and lower the pitch occasionally too, but retain the same note until it sends you gently to sleep.

TONIGHT'S TRIVIA

• In 1666 there was a great fire which completely destroyed half of London, but amazingly there were only six deaths.
• One Irish cure for mumps is to be led around a pigsty on reins.

- Iron nails cannot be used in oak wood because the acid in the wood would rust them in no time.
- The women of the Kirghiz tribe in Asia face divorce if they mention the name of their husband.

October 23

TONIGHT'S CURE

Remember when ...? Cast your mind back to a particular time or incident when you found it a great struggle to keep awake, but had to. Perhaps you had a particular assignment to complete, an exam to study for, or a journey to continue that made it impossible for you to stop and go to sleep, however badly you wished to. Do you remember how very hard it was to remain awake? Try to concentrate carefully on that situation, and then blot out what it was that kept you awake so that now there is nothing to prevent you from going to sleep, and you will soon drop off.

TONIGHT'S TRIVIA

- In the seventeenth century an idea for a submarine was suggested to the British admiralty, but it was dismissed on the grounds that it "would never work."
- All the continents, excluding Antarctica, are wider in the north than in the south.
- Having mated, the black widow spider then eats her husband.
- In Albuquerque, New Mexico, a waiter was admitted to the hospital suffering from burns after a flaming duck he was serving exploded.

October 24

TONIGHT'S CURE

Stop waiting. The worst thing you can do in bed at night is to lie and *wait* for sleep, because like the old proverb—a watched pot never boils—and that is the reason why so many cures divert your mind to enable you to sleep. So *stop* thinking how awful you will look in the morning. *Stop* thinking how tired you will be tomorrow. *Stop* reflecting on the bags under your eyes. Instead, think positively. Say, "Why the hell do I want to go to sleep anyway?" Think about how there really is no point in sleeping, it is an absolute waste of time, and how life is much too short already without spending a third of it asleep. If you think along these lines you'll be asleep before you can say, "I don't give a damn!"

• The windows of an empty house never frost over, no matter how low the temperature.

• The film star Greta Garbo once worked as a manicurist.

• In Ohio there is a law that animals out after dark must have reflective lights on their tails.

• The highest and lowest points in the lower forty-eight states are only eighty miles apart.

October 25

TONIGHT'S CURE

Q-cure. Tonight you're going to forget about twenty five letters of the alphabet and concentrate all your mental powers on just one letter. The cure known commonly as *Q* consists of taking that particular letter, visualizing it in your mind, and looking at the shape of it. Take a specific theme—place names, states, book titles, games, food, movie stars, etc.—and think of as many items in each category which begin with *Q*. If you exhaust all the possibilities, try using *X, Y,* and *Z*. I bet sleep will come before you ever reach *Z*.

TONIGHT'S TRIVIA

• Cicadas hear through their stomachs.

• When anyone died in Persia the mourners used to bottle their tears at the funeral in the belief that the liquid had healing properties.

• The entire population of Norway is only equal to one-third the number of people living in New Mexico.

• The Canadian river does not flow through Canada, or anywhere near it.

October 26

TONIGHT'S CURE

Samuel Coleridge. The most soporific lines of poetry ever written are said to be those of Samuel Taylor Coleridge. Repeat them to yourself over and over again tonight when you get into bed. Then turn out the light and try to remember them, and once you do. continue repeating them until you feel sleepy:

Oh sleep! it is a gentle thing
Beloved from pole to pole.
To Mary Queen the praise be given!

She sent the gentle sleep from Heaven,
That slid into my soul.

TONIGHT'S TRIVIA

• The death penalty is still enforced in Britain for anyone convicted of high treason.
• Trawlers catching fish use nets larger than a football field.
• In Fiji you need governmental permission to take whale teeth out of the country.
• In Minnesota it is illegal to hang male and female underwear on the same line.

October 27

TONIGHT'S CURE

Energetic breathtaking. Before getting into bed tonight, stand at an open window. Now close your eyes and breathe in very deeply, raising your arms up, across your body, up over your head, and back down to your sides as you breathe so your hands will have made a complete circle through the air. To keep the correct rhythm remember that your arms must go up as you inhale and down as you exhale. Now repeat this ten times before getting into bed.

TONIGHT'S TRIVIA

• In strict medical terms *morons* are more intelligent than *imbeciles*.
• Queen Elizabeth I did not possess any land outside England and Wales.
• Peas are the most widely eaten vegetable.
• Both the U.S. Navy and Theodore Roosevelt were born today. The Navy was established by the Continental Congress in 1775 and Roosevelt came into the world in 1858.

October 28

TONIGHT'S CURE

Bed is bed. The whole purpose of a bed is to sleep in it. If you do not sleep in your bed then it is being wrongly used. Therefore to treat your bed correctly and overcome your insomnia at the same time you should make a point of practicing the following. Go to bed at your usual time. Lie down and attempt to fall asleep. If you are not asleep in ten to fifteen minutes, then get up. Go and do something until you feel that you can sleep. Then return to bed. If you still do not sleep, get up again. Only get back in bed when you feel really tired. It could be that you will spend a complete night without any sleep. Do not worry, you will sleep the next night. However, if you reach a stage when you feel too tired to get out of bed again then you are tired enough to fall asleep.

TONIGHT'S TRIVIA

• The skull of a Zimbabwe man which is said to be forty thousand years old shows that he suffered from tooth decay.
• People who were born blind dream in sounds, not pictures.
• A duck is the only bird to have nostrils at the end of its beak.
• Two historic symbols of the United States came into being on October 28. Harvard College (as it then was called) was founded in 1636 and two hundred and fifty years later to the day the Statue of Liberty was dedicated, after being assembled from the 214 pieces which arrived from France.

October 29

TONIGHT'S CURE

Insomniac's club. If you know of a number of people who suffer from insomnia then why don't you form your own club? There are very few activities that you do during the day which cannot be done at night. Many people, especially city dwellers, do not like to wander outside alone at night, but they would if others joined them—and fresh air is really a great cure for insomnia. So go ahead and organize a midnight stroll or a midnight picnic at least one night a week. I am told that in New York there is a group called "Friends of the Parks" who go out on "insomniac bicycle tours" which are said to be very enjoyable owing to the lack of traffic and the participants are able to engage in pastimes that would otherwise be impossible to do during the day.

TONIGHT'S TRIVIA

• On the Caribbean island of Haiti buses are called tap-taps.
• Birds can occasionally set their own broken wings.
• There are more than one thousand different Arabic words for camel.
• Takers of sleeping pills dream less than those who do not take sleeping pills.

October 30

Red herring. As you will probably know, a red herring has nothing to do with fish; it is a false clue or something designed to mislead you. In our language we have many names of animals like this which do not exist, or lend their names to something different. For example, we know that in India the cow is sacred, but a sacred cow is something completely different. Think of a Scotch woodcock, the black sheep of the family, and the Welsh Rabbit you consume. Now see if you can think of at least ten more animals that are red herrings like these.

TONIGHT'S TRIVIA

• The first owner of the *Mona Lisa* hung it in his bathroom.
• The distance between the earth and the sun is over three-hundred eighty times greater than the distance between the earth and the moon.
• In Toronto, Canada, there is a church called the St. James Bond United Church. (Do you suppose they sing hymn number 007?)
• Napoleon Bonaparte designed the Italian flag.

October 31

TONIGHT'S CURE

Halloween cure. Tonight the ancient feast of Halloween is being celebrated the world over. This is the *Eve of All-Hallows* when witches are said to fly through the sky on broomsticks, and when all the demons and goblins prowl the face of the earth. Imagine that you are a good witch tonight, one that can only cast good spells. Among your many powers you have the ability to fly anywhere in the world, and on this special night you must travel far and wide to cast ten good spells. Given this power, what good would you do in the world tonight? Choose carefully, ten spells is your maximum and there's a lot to occupy you tonight!

TONIGHT'S TRIVIA

• In the sixteenth century witches could be distinguished by their habit of throwing back their hair, an inability to cry, and their practice of walking backward intertwining their fingers.
• On the eve of Alexander the Great's expedition into Asia, a statue of Orpheus is reported to have sweated profusely.
• Harry Houdini, the great escapologist who had enough tricks to

fill any witch's cauldron, died on October 31, 1926. He had lapsed into a coma some days before, but when he finally died, some friends commented that he hung on in order to make a good headline.

• Los Angeles has five-hundred thousand more automobiles than people.

November 1

TONIGHT'S CURE

Almanac cure. Having reached this far in the *Insomniac's Almanac* you will now have had the opportunity to experience 305 different cures to date, a list which now provides you with a cure of its very own. When you get to bed tonight, without cheating by looking back in the book, make a list of fifty names of any cures that have been described so far. Then if you're still awake, put into practice whichever one you found to be most effective.

TONIGHT'S TRIVIA

• Among the many curious sights revealed by X rays is one of a five-hundred-thousand-year-old piece of rock which appears to have a modern spark plug at its core.

• A slice of lemon has been served with fish since the Middle Ages, not just for the taste, but lemon was believed to dissolve any bones you may have swallowed.

• Asses and horses clean themselves by rolling in the dust.

• In Sweden there is a town called Å.

November 2

TONIGHT'S CURE

Escape. Leave the cares of the world and the aches and pains of daily life behind you tonight, and take a trip to the trouble-free world outside your body. Start by lying completely flat on your back, without a pillow. Make sure that the room is totally dark. Close your eyes and start breathing deeply for a count of fifty. Feel your body relaxing muscle by muscle, from your toes to your head. Become aware of the rhythm of your breathing until it lulls you into a state of total peace. Now leave your body behind, forget all about it and escape to that distant other world. Forget completely about your body, forget all your problems associated with it. Raise your eyes to look up under your eyelids and make your mind a complete blank, and then give your spirit free rein to wander where it will.

TONIGHT'S TRIVIA

- American Indians used to smoke pipes through their noses.
- Boxwood sinks in water.
- The original Cinderella was an Egyptian.
- Glen Miller's hit "Chattanooga Choo Choo" was the first to be awarded a gold disc for selling over one million copies.

November 3

TONIGHT'S CURE

Embryonic sleep. Have you ever wondered what it would be like to be enclosed in a shell like a baby bird? How warm and reassuring it would be, and how dark. After you turn out your light tonight, pretend that you are in your shell, warm and snug, protected from the world outside, isolated in your own cozy darkness. Now curl up tightly in a ball and enjoy the comforting protection that you have tonight.

TONIGHT'S TRIVIA

- In 1959, 53 million ball point pens were sold in the United Kingdom alone.
- The seventeenth King of Poland, John III, was born, crowned, married, and died on the same day of the same month.
- The planet Uranus can be seen by the naked eye.
- Hawaii grows over a third of the world's pineapples.

November 4

TONIGHT'S CURE

Tension release. As we have already discovered, much of the tension that keeps us awake is located in and around the eyes. Fortunately there is a simple technique to release this tension. Begin by closing your eyes tightly. Now raise your eyebrows and wrinkle up your forehead, holding this position for at least one minute, and then relax—noticing how different it feels. Now screw up your eyes very tightly and again hold for at least one minute before relaxing them. Now wrinkle up your nose, hold that for one minute, and relax. Repeat this cycle by wrinkling up your forehead, then your eyes, and finally your nose. Repeat this continuously until you feel that the tension has dissipated.

TONIGHT'S TRIVIA

• Britain's George IV used to maintain his complexion by being bled daily.
• Early golf balls were made of leather and stuffed with feathers.
• The first U.S. colonies in 1610 had a grand total of 350 people.
• The forerunner of one of the world's most lethal weapons, the Gatling gun, was patented by its inventor on November 4, 1862. And on the same date, ninety years later, President Harry Truman made another advance in U.S. security when he founded the National Security Agency.

November 5

· ·

TONIGHT'S CURE

Sleep centers. If you are a chronic insomniac, and there are hundreds of Americans who are, you might find a visit to one of the numerous sleep centers located throughout the country very rewarding. Here scientists researching the reasons why people cannot sleep will set out to find why *you* cannot sleep and they'll decide what is the most effective method of remedying your complaint. The first sleep center was established in California at Stanford University, and the second was opened in the East at Montefiore Hospital in New York. Later the Association of Sleep Disorder Centers was set up in Cincinnati. Now there are centers all over the United States and Canada where you'll find trained staff fully equipped to deal with *your* problem to help you find a cure. So make enquiries today, or if today's almost gone, go to sleep, confident in the knowledge that tomorrow many of your problems could be solved.

TONIGHT'S TRIVIA

• At the end of the nineteenth century many doctors believed that chewing gum would exhaust your salivary glands.
• Only white bread is used during a Holy Communion.
• John Cage, an American composer, composed a piece of music called *"4'33"* " (four minutes and thirty-three seconds) in which not a single note is played.
• Both President Grover Cleveland and his chief political opponent, James G. Blaine, were draft dodgers.

November 6

TONIGHT'S CURE

Shipwreck. Tonight you have a chance to play Robinson Crusoe—
but on your own terms. Imagine you have foreknowledge that you
are going to be shipwrecked on a beautiful tropical island. Given
this knowledge, plan exactly what you would wish to have with you
when cast ashore. And, as there will be only one other survivor,
decide who you would most like to have with you. Your choice can
be as extravagant or outlandish as you like. However, your
companion must be alive at present and remember that you might
have to spend the rest of your days together!

TONIGHT'S TRIVIA

• A noise of 210 decibels could bore a hole in a piece of wood.
• When you board a boat in Spain you must put your right foot on
first for good luck.
• The triangle is a symbol of a happy marriage in Greece.
• In the eighteenth century Jonathan Swift and Samuel Johnson
wanted to ban several words, including stingy, clever, bully,
bamboozle, mob, and banter.

November 7

TONIGHT'S CURE

Lunchtime snooze. Contrary as it may seem, many insomniacs
benefit from a siesta during the day and doctors agree that one of
the best times for this siesta is right after lunch. Even if you simply
rest your head on your desk at work for half an hour and do not
sleep, the effect will be very refreshing. However, never have more
than one-and-a-half hours sleep during the day as this will make
you feel sluggish. A one-half to one-hour nap will make you feel
refreshed, relaxed, and better equipped to face the remainder of
the day. As a result you will take a lot less time to unwind in the
evening and will sleep much more soundly when you go to bed.

TONIGHT'S TRIVIA

• Moslems wear white at funerals.
• Long-tailed sheep in Asia Minor pull small trolleys behind them
to support their tails.
• A butterfly looks at you with twelve thousand eyes.
• Ronald Hamilton of western Australia carried a 105-pound brick
in his ungloved hand for 40 miles.

November 8

TONIGHT'S CURE

Back cure. If you are one of the millions of people who suffer from a slight backache during the night, especially when there is a drop in temperature, then you can perform the following cure to help you sleep. First check to make sure that your mattress is firm enough to support you correctly and it is not that which is causing your trouble. Start the cure before going to bed by taking a warm bath, though not a very hot one as that can be bad for your spine. Before you get in add a tablespoon of cooking salt to the water. Soak in this water for no longer than five minutes, then gently pat yourself dry. Take a hot-water bottle to bed wrapped in a towel or small blanket. Place it against your back at the point where it usually aches. This should stop any stiffness and give you an undisturbed night's sleep.

TONIGHT'S TRIVIA

• Dentists extract ten tons of rotten teeth from American children annually.
• The lunar year has 354 days.
• The North American tarantula has a bite as harmful as a pin prick.
• A shark's skeleton contains no bones.

November 9

• •

TONIGHT'S CURE

State banquet. While you may not be indulging your body with sleep at present, here's a cure which will at least let you indulge it with food and wine, if only in your mind. Pretend that you have been invited to a state banquet at the White House. Also pretend that you are allowed to choose your own menu. There are to be ten separate courses and your appetite during the evening will be limitless, so plan exactly what you would like to eat and drink drawing on all the exotic and diverse culinary talents the world has to offer. Will you limit your menu to foods from one country? Or will you take the best of ten national menus? The choice is yours.

TONIGHT'S TRIVIA

• One Louise Elizabeth Vaughan gave birth to five nuns, three priests, two bishops, and a cardinal.

- Over thirty states in the United States produce gasoline.
- Ancient Greeks used the ankle bones of sheep to make dice.
- The Great Fire of Boston broke out on November 9, 1872, the same date on which the redoubtable actress Katharine Hepburn was born in Hartford, Connecticut, in 1909.

November 10

TONIGHT'S CURE

Trivia cure. Having now been given well over twelve hundred exciting pieces of trivia over the last year you should be able to remember some of it, even if it is only things like the spider's penis is on the end of its foot and Jayne Mansfield's bust measurement. Hopefully more will have been retained than you imagine. Close this book, turn out the light, and remember at least fifty amazing facts from *Tonight's Trivia* before you even think about going to sleep. Here are four to start you off on tonight's cure.

TONIGHT'S TRIVIA

- William Buckland, a nineteenth century dean of Westminster, ate Louis XIV's embalmed heart at dinner one evening.
- Bloomers are named after Mrs. Amelia Jenks Bloomer who first wore them in New York, in 1851.
- In the ancient world sneezing was a favorable omen.
- When a census was taken among Eskimos fewer than one in forty-six had ever seen an igloo.

November 11

TONIGHT'S CURE

Parachute. Imagine that you have just jumped from a plane several thousand feet in the air and are parachuting down to safety. Pull your rip cord and just let yourself drift in the breeze. There is nothing you can do, or need do, so just relax as you float down and down and down into a deep, deep sleep. Feel the gentle swinging motion of the parachute and you may be asleep by the time you reach the ground.

TONIGHT'S TRIVIA

- A piece of glass cracks when moving at twenty-five hundred miles per hour.

- Over 95 percent of fifteen-year-olds have already developed some permanent decay in their teeth.
- Walking uses eight times as much energy as writing.
- Fiery U.S. General George S. Patton was born in 1885 on November 11, the day on which the firing stopped all over Europe at the end of World War I. (The war ended at the eleventh hour of the eleventh day of the eleventh month.)

November 12

TONIGHT'S CURE

Tug-of-war. Tonight, when you're lying in bed unable to sleep, don't try to convince yourself that you're not uptight when you really are. Instead try to increase your tension in active competition. Picture yourself in a tug-of-war with a strong opponent. Feel the rope biting into your hands as you tighten your grip. Feel your legs bursting and straining as you try to take a step back. Be aware of the pressure on every muscle in your body as you fight to make ground without losing an inch. Now suddenly feel your opponent give way. At first you'll just feel a loosening of the tension. But this will be followed by a wonderful freedom that will send you rolling over on your back as you fall away, loose and relaxed, after your exertions. And afterwards just lie stretched out in the grass enjoying the peace and quiet after the struggle.

TONIGHT'S TRIVIA

- Until recently prisoners condemned to death in Mongolia were nailed into coffins and left on the steppe.
- In England oak trees are struck by lightning more frequently than any other type of tree.
- The word *tragedy* comes from the Greek word meaning Goat Song.
- Domestic gas is odorless in its natural state; it is given a smell so that leaks can be detected.

November 13

TONIGHT'S CURE

Diet analysis. One major cause of insomnia can be either a vitamin deficiency or a lack of sufficient minerals. Our bodies are like a car or a piece of machinery—if they do not receive the right ingredients and energy supply, they will not work, or will only give very poor performance. So check your diet, as you lie awake tonight, to make sure that you are getting enough protein from milk, eggs, meat, and dairy products. (Calcium and carbohydrates are important too, plus a certain amount of roughage to ensure regular bowel movement as constipation can also cause insomnia.) If you feel there may be something lacking in your daily intake, take a course of multivitamin and iron pills to supplement your diet. This is not an instant cure, but over the next two weeks you will start to feel healthier and you'll find some improvement in your sleeping habits. (Your doctor, or a sleep center, will give you a list of foods that you should and should not eat.)

TONIGHT'S TRIVIA

• The religious practice of kissing the Pope's toe lasted for over one thousand years until it was abolished in 1773.

• People did not start eating three meals a day until a century ago.

• Oysters should not be eaten in a month that does not contain the letter *R*.

• The word *onion* means large pearl.

November 14
....

TONIGHT'S CURE

Wedding day. Focus your attention on past good times tonight. Think back to one of the most important days in any person's life—their wedding day. Think back to the day you were married, or the day you attended the wedding of a friend or close relative. Can you remember the beauty of the service, the hymns that were sung, and what people were wearing? Can you remember each of the guests? Can you remember the wedding feast, what was eaten and what was said? And if today happens to be your own wedding anniversary, you and your partner should share a bottle of champagne in bed tonight and pretend it is your honeymoon—it's the best cure for insomnia.

TONIGHT'S TRIVIA

• When Princess Anne and Captain Mark Phillips were married on November 14, 1973, her bouquet contained a sprig of myrtle grown from a myrtle used in Queen Victoria's wedding bouquet.

• Bachelors are twice as susceptible to disease as married men.

• Women of Togoland, Africa, wear a small bustle of straw to show their married status.

• Over five-hundred thousand Americans died of influenza in 1918.

November 15

TONIGHT'S CURE

——lyn. You may have tried to cure your insomnia by thinking about girls before. But this cure's different. What you have to do is think of as many girls' names as you can that end in *lyn*. You might be surprised at how many there are. Start with Marilyn and Carolyn, and see if you can find at least twenty more before you attempt to fall asleep tonight.

TONIGHT'S TRIVIA

• A frog's tongue grows from the front of its mouth.
• In 1776 the British government offered £5,000 to anyone who could find the Northwest Passage.
• The French Empress and wife of Napoleon, Marie Louise, could move her ears at will and even turn them inside out.
• Hindu babies do not have their nails cut until after their first birthday.

November 16

TONIGHT'S CURE

Abstinence. If you're awake at the moment and unable to get to sleep make a resolution for tomorrow. Throughout the day abstain from two things—caffeine and sugar. Get through the entire day without touching one drop of coffee, so that by the time you go to bed it will be at least twenty-four hours since you drank any. Cut down as much as possible on substances that contain sugar. Do without sugary cereals, biscuits or pastries, candies or cakes, and sugared drinks. Artificial sweeteners such as saccharin may be used if essential, but try to be strong-willed. If you can be you will lower your blood sugar and thereby cut out a major stimulant, which combined with the caffeine in large quantities could be preventing you from sleep.

TONIGHT'S TRIVIA

• A sea horse can grasp objects with its tail.
• British lawyers still wear black in court as a sign of mourning for William III's wife, Queen Mary, who died in 1664.
• Every ninety seconds someone in the United States dies of cancer.
• A whip cracks because it is moving faster than the speed of sound.

November 17

TONIGHT'S CURE

Vegetable juice. Vegetable juice has been proven to be a great tonic for people suffering from insomnia and it is advisable for insomniacs to drink two glasses a day—one in the morning and one at night. Vegetable juice can be purchased bottled or canned, but if you have your own blender or juice extractor you can experiment with different vegetables and have a much greater variety. Doctors recommend celery and carrot juice. Take about nine ounces of each of these and mix them together. Personal preference might make you decide to have more carrot juice than celery juice or vice versa. Whichever you choose, it's sure to do you good.

TONIGHT'S TRIVIA

• Two great literary figures who we hold in high esteem are Socrates and Homer, although we have none of their actual writings that we can read.

• A snail's teeth are on the edge of its tongue, which it uses like a knife.

• There is a particular species of butterfly in Brazil which is brown in color and smells of chocolate.

• On reentering the earth's atmosphere the space shuttle reaches temperatures of 10,832° F.

November 18

TONIGHT'S CURE

Laughter. Laughter is one of the greatest muscle relaxers known to man. One eminent British doctor I spoke to recommended that the best way to relieve tension and have a good night's sleep is to go and see a good comic play or watch a comic movie. He felt that a few good belly laughs with the Marx Brothers or a chuckle while watching a farce would do more for a person than any pill ever invented. So get all the laughter you can this evening. Go and see a very light movie or invite over some entertaining friends whom you know are always good for a laugh. Then go all out to have a good time and you'll have a good night's sleep as a bonus.

TONIGHT'S TRIVIA

• Julius Caesar wore a laurel wreath to disguise the fact that he was bald.

- The whalebones used in corsets came from a whale's mouth.
- If a lump of ice is wrapped in enough glass fibre it can be baked in an oven without melting.
- On the day the talking Mickey Mouse was officially born (November 18, 1928), the United States also celebrated the birthday of Standard Time (1883) and the signing of the Panama Canal Treaty with Panama (1903).

November 19

TONIGHT'S CURE

Fruits. Take a world tour tonight through nature's larder and make a mental list, in alphabetical order, of every fruit you can think of that can be found around the world. Start with *A* for apples, *B* for bananas, *C* for crabapples, and continue through to *Z*. Then when you've completed the list, repeat it in reverse order from *Z* to *A*.

TONIGHT'S TRIVIA

- Leaves on a eucalyptus tree hang vertically.
- To test if an object is really gold place it in nitric acid. If the object is not gold it will turn green.
- The Median prophet Zoroaster lived entirely on cheese for thirty years.
- A ten-gallon hat holds six pints.

November 20

TONIGHT'S CURE

Le mot juste. The influence of many cultures on our language has resulted in the inclusion of many foreign words and phrases that we use in our everyday speech without a second thought. We say things are *passe,* talk of *billet doux* and *belles lettres,* say people are *bourgeois,* and churn out phrases like *nil desperandum* and *mutatis mutandis* at the drop of a hat. So tonight, take a sheet of paper and write down as many foreign words and phrases as you can think of that are in common usage today. If it makes it easier, do this from *A* to *Z*.

TONIGHT'S TRIVIA

- Figures show that more people are killed after being kicked by donkeys than are killed in plays.

- Real diamonds always feel cold, imitations do not.
- In Cuba it is believed to be dangerous to walk around in moonlight without a hat.
- Cyanide poison can be made from apple seeds.

November 21

TONIGHT'S CURE

Why worry? If there is a particular worry preventing you from sleeping tonight, think back to a past trouble and see how you rode that storm and survived. Reassure yourself with the knowledge that there is no tragedy too big to handle. Franklin D. Roosevelt once said that fear stems from fear itself. Obviously you cannot be happy all the time, but always try to get your worries into perspective by remembering that nothing is so great that it cannot be solved and nothing is worth losing any sleep over.

TONIGHT'S TRIVIA

- King Alphonse of Spain was one of the few people to be born a king.
- Every tenth egg is larger than the preceding nine.
- Millionaire Paul Getty once wrote a book entitled *How To Be Rich.*
- The famous eighteenth century commander, General Blucher, lived in permanent fear of giving birth to an elephant.

November 22

TONIGHT'S CURE

Position. Could it be that there's something wrong with the way in which you're trying to sleep? Are you lying as comfortably as you can? Tonight experiment by changing the position in which you sleep. If you normally sleep on your right side try changing to the left. If you sleep on your stomach then attempt to sleep on your back. See if your new position helps you breathe more easily. See if it's one that you can remain in comfortably all night. You might find that it takes you a night or two to get used to the change, but many people have found that it's well worth the effort.

TONIGHT'S TRIVIA

- Pouring hot water into a glass is more likely to crack it if the glass is thick than if it is thin.

- The human body contains enough potassium to explode a toy cannon.
- When electric batteries were first invented people feared they would explode.
- In China the sign of a cross indicates a porn shop.

November 23

TONIGHT'S CURE

Eye relaxation. The moment you turn out your light tonight close your eyes and screw your eyelids up very tightly. Don't move your head at all, but look up with your eyes still tightly closed. Hold this position for forty-five seconds concentrating on maintaining the tension. Then let your eyelids and your eyes relax completely for five full minutes. Now repeat the exercise but this time look down as you screw up your eyelids. Again hold this for forty-five seconds and then relax for another five minutes. When you repeat this the third time look to the left before relaxing your gaze and finally look to the right, before relaxing your eyes completely and falling asleep.

TONIGHT'S TRIVIA

- One early governor of New York was a notorious transvestite and even wore female clothes for his official portrait.
- Giuseppe Verdi's opera *Aida* was written to commemorate the opening of the Suez Canal.
- Spiders are used in the manufacture of anaesthetics.
- If all the frankfurters manufactured annually in the United States were joined end to end they would stretch to the moon and back two-and-a-half times.

November 24

TONIGHT'S CURE

Both ends. Tonight's cure offers you an alphabetical word game with a difference. It's one that you can do either with a pencil and paper or in your head. The aim is to think of words that begin and end with the same letter. Start with *A* for *alpha* and work your way through to *Z* for...? (If you're lucky it might be Zzzzzz....)

TONIGHT'S TRIVIA

- In China a doctor used to hang a lantern outside his house for

every one of his patients that died.
- Immediately after a bee stings you, it dies.
- Some flowers, such as crocuses, have been known to force their way through tarmac.
- In August, 1972, there were thirteen murders in New York City every day.

November 25

TONIGHT'S CURE

Baseball game. You know the hypnotic effect that watching a tennis ball zipping back and forth over a net can have. Well the same effect can help you get to sleep at night. Once you're in bed tonight, close your eyes and start thinking about a ball game you have watched. You can choose any game you like; baseball, racquet ball, tennis, even soccer. The game itself isn't important, nor is the score. You just have to fixate your eyes on the ball all the time. Watch it hurtle around the court or flash across the field and never lose sight of it. After a while you'll start to feel the hypnotic effect and after that—you'll be asleep.

TONIGHT'S TRIVIA

- Aborigines treated wounds with mold from trees thousands of years before penicillin was discovered.
- Roscoe Tanner can serve a tennis ball at 140 miles an hour.
- During the reign of Edward III, in England, it was against the law to eat more than two meals a day.
- The muscles of the human jaw exert a force of 590 pounds.

November 26

TONIGHT'S CURE

Novel experience. Tonight you have the chance to discover if there really is a novel inside you. If you're lying awake, unable to sleep, use the time to get to work on your masterpiece. Start by working out the plot. It's going to be twenty chapters long, so you'll need to work out exactly what's going to happen in each chapter. Who are your main characters going to be? What will each of them be like? Are you going to model them on friends or are they going to be total strangers? Once you've organized that in your mind you'll have to decide on the title. Then, if you wake up in the night, start the first paragraph.

- The Sphinx is a statue of the goddess Armachis.
- Film stars used to wear sunglasses to relieve their eyes from the dazzle of the powerful studio lights.
- The hairs of a man's beard are as strong as copper wire of the same thickness.
- The full name of the chemical tryptophan synthetase, whose chemical formula is $C_{1289}H_{2051}N_{343}O_{375}S_8$, has 1,913 letters.

November 27

TONIGHT'S CURE

Four minus four. If big numbers exhaust you just thinking about them try this cure to send you to sleep this evening.

When you get to bed, turn out the light and close your eyes. Start with number four thousand and count backwards in fours until you reach one. (Most people rarely reach three thousand before they are asleep.)

TONIGHT'S TRIVIA

- In Russia there are one hundred women for every eighty-five men.
- A great proportion of women develop bunions before they reach the age of forty.
- In India there are 114 hymns dedicated to the soma plant.
- Studies in cannibalism reveal that a man weighing one-hundred fifty pounds would feed seventy-five people.

November 28

TONIGHT'S CURE

Energy consumption. If you can't get to sleep because your body feels restless and full of go, then how about making everything you do tomorrow as energetic as possible? Try not to keep still for one minute. Jog to work, or at the very least jog to the bus stop. At work never use the elevator if you can use the stairs. Spend as much time on your feet as you can while at work. Go for a walk at lunchtime even if it is only around the block. When you get home, do all those energetic jobs around the house, such as housework and washing the car. Then in the evening do not sit in front of the TV but go to a dance, involve yourself in a sport of some kind, or go for a bike ride. And last thing at night go for a late night walk before you go to bed. You're sure to feel worn out when bedtime comes, and, who knows, you could alter your whole life-style too!

TONIGHT'S TRIVIA

• Queen Elizabeth II was born in a private house with a street number.
• A pint of vinegar is heavier in winter than in summer.
• Insomniacs move as much as one hundred times in one night.
• From the time you are a baby to the time you reach adulthood your eyes only increase three and one-quarter times in size.

November 29

TONIGHT'S CURE

Hot broth. There's an old New England remedy for insomnia which tells you to drink a bowl or cup of hot beef broth before retiring to bed. This will warm you, relax you, and nourish you, the cure claims. You can make your own broth by boiling bones with chopped vegetables and making your own stock. Alternatively you can buy it conveniently in a can, but if you do, buy a brand that is thick and contains real meat and vegetables. The only other point to remember is that you should drink this half an hour before you go to bed.

TONIGHT'S TRIVIA

• Rats can survive longer without water than camels.
• The dormouse spends six months in hibernation.
• Shakespeare coined seventeen hundred words, including monumental, laughable, leapfrog, gnarled, hurry, castigate, barefaced, and auspicious.
• The Red Sea is never mentioned by name in the Bible.

November 30

TONIGHT'S CURE

Shoulder stand. Among the many yoga positions designed to help you relax and unwind this one works well to increase the flow of blood to your head, shoulders, and neck. Begin by lying on your back, flat on the floor, palms downward, and breathing deeply. Now stiffen your stomach muscles and raise your hips with your hands. Straighten your body slowly with your legs pointing upward, and put your weight on the back of your shoulders and the back of your head, with the rest of your body pointing upright. Check that your arms form a triangle with your body. Now press your chin against your chest so that the entire weight of your body is supported by your shoulders and your arms. Hold this position for one minute and then slowly relax. Have a short rest and then repeat this three times before you get into bed.

TONIGHT'S TRIVIA

- George Washington carried a portable sundial instead of a watch.
- Bears take hot sulphur baths to ease the pain of growing old.
- George Frederick Handel wrote many of his operas for eunuchs, which helps to explain why they are seldom performed today.
- The opposite sides of a die always add up to eight.

December 1

TONIGHT'S CURE

Shall I compare thee to a summer's day? As winter draws nigh, cast your mind back to a warm summer's day. Not just any summer's day, but one specific memorable day last summer that was particularly enjoyable and which stands out in your mind. Perhaps it was a visit to the beach, a family picnic, a long walk through a park, or a day hiking. It doesn't matter what it was, or what you did, so long as it was something that brings back happy memories. Once you've picked your day, lie back and remember the warmth and the good time you had that day.

TONIGHT'S TRIVIA

- On the Isle of Sark in the English Channel there is a prison that holds a maximum of two prisoners.
- Gioacchino Rossini wrote the *Barber of Seville* in eight days.
- In heraldic terminology the *stars* and *stripes* should be *mullets* and *barrulets*.
- Woody Allen was born on December 1, 1935, the day on which Jolly Irene fell out of bed in Coney Island two years later. People fall out of bed all the time of course. What made Irene special was that it took five men to lift her back into bed again. Jolly Irene was the Ringling Brothers' famous fat lady and she weighed 650 pounds!

December 2

TONIGHT'S CURE

Four poster. Until the nineteenth century many people slept in a four-poster bed, and having slept in one, I can tell you that they have very great advantages for the insomniac. They are completely dark inside once the curtains are closed, and they are free from any drafts. They keep you warm, safe, and secure inside, far away from all the worries, hustle, and bustle of the outside world and they give you total privacy. If you want to see whether you like them it is possible to construct a temporary four poster of your own by erecting a pole at each of the four corners of your bed, throwing one blanket over the top to make a canopy, and attaching others to the sides to make curtains. Try spending tonight in your own four poster and if you sleep well, you may want to invest in a genuine antique.

TONIGHT'S TRIVIA

• On the night the Dead Sea Scrolls were deciphered for the first time, the United Nations voted in favor of granting Israel statehood.
• King Saul was the first reported person to have committed suicide by falling on his sword.
• The word *Amen* is Hebrew for So be it.
• The Atomic Age was born in a disused squash court in Chicago when the world's first atomic pile, constructed by scientists from Columbia and Princeton, started geiger counters clicking.

December 3

TONIGHT'S CURE

The Paul James nightcap. This is a delicious, original, and effective remedy for insomnia and you will soon be drinking it every night. Place a large cupful of milk in a saucepan and bring it to a boil. If you have a sweet tooth, add some golden syrup or honey and stir it around while the milk simmers. Now add two or three drops of peppermint extract and three teaspoonfuls of instant cocoa powder or drinking chocolate. Continue stirring the mixture as it simmers until it becomes thick and creamy. Then pour it back into your cup, sprinkle a little grated cinnamon on the top, add a marshmallow or a spoonful of cream to the surface, and sip it slowly to enjoy it fully. (If you want you can add a few drops of rum or brandy just before you drink it.)

TONIGHT'S TRIVIA

• In China, eggs are buried in the ground for three months before they are eaten, in order to "ripen" them.
• King Gustav III, of Sweden, was convinced that coffee was a

poison and sentenced one condemned criminal to drink it until he died. The man lived to be eighty-three years old.
- The question mark developed from cutting a *q* for question.
- Tin cans are 97 percent steel.

December 4

TONIGHT'S CURE

Christmas presents. How about getting well ahead with holiday shopping this year? If you're awake tonight, start planning your holiday gift list. It will be a weight off your mind later on and the exercise for your brain will soon tire you. Take a sheet of paper and write down on the left-hand side the names of each person with whom you exchange presents. If possible, jot down what you bought that person last year so you do not repeat the gift. Then write down a suggestion for at least one present per person until you feel sleepy. If you are still awake, try to estimate how much each is going to cost, then you can decide when and where to make the purchases.

TONIGHT'S TRIVIA

- A nineteenth century composer, Louis Jullien, had thirty-six Christian names.
- In 1971, astronaut Alan Shepherd hit a golf ball four hundred yards across the surface of the moon.
- A medium-sized swarm of locusts, numbering about one million, can devour twenty tons of food a day.
- In 1922 a twenty-four-year-old woman pleaded guilty to sixty-one bigamous marriages.

December 5

TONIGHT'S CURE

Head and shoulders. Although few of us realize it, one of the most common reasons for insomnia is that our heads and shoulders are exposed to cold drafts at night. This explains why old fashioned nightcaps are suddenly coming back into fashion after a long absence, because if your head is warm, then the rest of your body will be warm. We lose a tremendous amount of heat from the top of our head, about 40 percent, so a nightcap seems like a good idea. If you do not have a nightcap, you can simply place a shawl or scarf very lightly over your head and shoulders, as long as it does not restrict your breathing in any way or give you a feeling of claustrophobia. If you sleep well tonight as a result, perhaps you should take a leaf out of your great-grandfather's book, and start wearing a nightcap regularly.

TONIGHT'S TRIVIA

• At the age of ninety our hearts pump about half as fast as they did when we were twenty.

• Venus rotates clockwise. All other planets rotate in a counter-clockwise direction.

• A pythoness is a witch, not a female snake.

• President Martin van Buren was born on December 5, 1782. He shares his birthday with General George Custer, born in 1839, and with Walt Disney, born in 1901. December 5, 1933, probably has even greater significance for most Americans, though, since that was the day on which Prohibition was repealed.

December 6

TONIGHT'S CURE

"The" Bible. If you've found all the trivia included so far enjoyable why not try compiling some of your own?

Take a copy of a Bible to bed with you tonight. It really does not matter which version you choose, just start at Genesis, Chapter 1, Verse 1, and begin to count how many times the word *the* appears. Get as far as you can before you feel sleepy, then put a marker in the page with a note of the total so far, and continue another night. You may eventually be able to find out exactly how many times *the* appears in the whole Bible—your very own trivia for tonight. Of course if you're really ambitious you could pick a whole list of words and count those at the same time. (Here's a few gems to encourage you.)

TONIGHT'S TRIVIA

• The word *Lord* occurs 1,855 times in the Bible. The words *reverend* and *girl* occur only once.

• No more than 6,654 words are used in all the books of the Bible and Talmud together.

• The Bible contains 66 Books, 1,189 chapters, and 33,173 verses.

• The nineteenth chapter of Kings II and the thirty-seventh chapter of Isaiah are almost identical.

December 7

TONIGHT'S CURE

Sight without sound. Do you fall asleep in front of the TV at night? If you do here's a TV cure with a difference. All you need is a TV in your bedroom. Maybe there's one there already? If there isn't, can you fix one up without too much difficulty? If you can sit up in bed with the lights out and the TV on turn down the volume completely, and watch the picture very carefully. The cure works best with stationary people such as newscasters and those being interviewed. However, any actors will do if there are no suitable programs available. Your concern isn't with the action anyway, because tonight you've got to concentrate on the mouths of the people on the screen. You've got to lip-read what they're saying and if you've never done it before, it will soon tire you out.

TONIGHT'S TRIVIA

• There are over five hundred characters in Tolstoy's *War and Peace.*

• Joseph Stalin only smoked a pipe in public. In private he chain-smoked cigarettes.

• Johann Georg Krünitz wrote an encyclopedia of 242 volumes, writing it entirely in long hand.

• The United States declared war on Austria-Hungary on December 7, 1917, which by a strange coincidence was the very day on which the Japanese attacked Pearl Harbor twenty-four years later.

December 8

TONIGHT'S CURE

What a state. Tonight you've got a chance to test your national geography. Take a sheet of paper to bed with you. Once you're in bed, and without looking at a map, draw an outline of the United States and attempt to fill in and name all the individual states. Try and complete the whole map unless you feel too tired to do so, which is the aim of the cure. You can check your accuracy in the morning.

TONIGHT'S TRIVIA

• Queen termites can lay eggs for up to fifty years.

• The U.S. mint once made the unfortunate error of stamping In Gold We Trust on a batch of coins instead of In God We Trust.

- People in their fifties tend to sleep less than those in their twenties, but people in their sixties get more sleep than at any time since childhood.
- A great step forward in the feminist movement was made by an unnamed actress on December 8, 1660. She became the first actress ever to appear on an English stage.

December 9

TONIGHT'S CURE

Digest readers. If you can't get to sleep tonight, or you've woken in the middle of the night, take a copy of the *Readers Digest* or a similar periodical. Go to the bathroom and *stand* there reading the magazine for at least thirty minutes. Then you can return to bed and should fall asleep almost immediately.

TONIGHT'S TRIVIA

- In 1631 an awkward error was made in one thousand copies of the Bible. Embarrassingly the word *not* was omitted from the seventh commandment, resulting in Thou Shalt Commit Adultery.
- One sixth of the land on earth is the USSR.
- The hummingbird can only use its feet for perching, it cannot walk.
- A snake in the London zoo was once fitted with an artificial eye.

December 10

TONIGHT'S CURE

Goldberg variations. In the 18th century, Johann Sebastian Bach composed the Goldberg variations for a young prince who was suffering from severe insomnia. On hearing the piece for the first time the Prince was lulled into a very deep sleep and it cured his sleep problem. Today, Bach's piece is available both on record and cassette and can be obtained also as a piano solo for those who find it more soothing. Keep a recording by your bed and send yourself to sleep with it whenever you find yourself staying awake.

TONIGHT'S TRIVIA

- In our language we use a vocabulary of a mere two thousand words to express most of what we wish to say.
- There is a point in the body in which acupuncture needles can be inserted to cure nymphomania and alcoholism.

- Dumbbells were originally bells with their clappers removed.
- In 1638 one Bishop Godwin described the sense of weightlessness on the moon.

December 11

Mattress turn. One of the most obvious reasons for insomnia is sheet discomfort caused by mattresses. Could this be the reason why you are kept awake? When you make your bed today, try removing all the bedclothes, then turn the mattress over and turn it from end-to-end also so the "foot" is now the "head." It might be a good idea to vacuum it thoroughly too before you remake the bed. The mattress is of vital importance to the way we sleep, and if not treated correctly the springs become worn and give little support. It might be an idea to invest in a new one if your own mattress is very old. This might be expensive of course, but what price can you put on a good night's sleep? Buy a good quality mattress with a long guarantee (federal regulations insist that each mattress has a guarantee). Check for support and comfort rather than attractiveness; after all, you are going to *feel* it more than you are going to *see* it.

TONIGHT'S TRIVIA

- There is no evidence to prove that mumps can cause sterility.
- Mao Tse-Tung was once a librarian.
- Leather has enough nutritional value to keep you alive in times when no food is available.
- The ancient Egyptians believed the world was hatched from an egg.

December 12

TONIGHT'S CURE

Celery cure. Put some sticks of celery in a glass or jug of water beside your bed when you go to sleep tonight. Then if you wake up in the night eat a stick, being sure to chew each mouthful twenty to thirty times. Celery is excellent for dieters too because it is one of the rare foods where you burn far more calories eating it than the celery itself actually contains. And in terms of insomnia, you should get so bored chewing away that you'll pretty soon fall back asleep again.

- By the year 2000 Yale University library will contain over 200 million books.
- The rings around Saturn are about fifty thousand miles in circumference, but only one foot thick.
- Pirates wore earrings to improve their eyesight, in the same way as acupuncturists insert a needle in the ear lobe to control senses in the eye.
- Our brains use one-fifth of the oxygen we inhale.

December 13

TONIGHT'S CURE

Greeting-card list. If you have not already done so, tonight is a good time to compile your greeting-card list, and even write your cards if you have them handy. Sit up in bed, take a sheet of paper, and write down every single person to whom you usually send a card. On average we receive roughly the same number each year, so if you know you generally receive fifty two, then write down the numbers one to fifty two on the left-hand side of the page and put a name against each number. Once you have compiled the list you can begin writing your cards until you feel sleepy, and you can fall asleep with the virtuous knowledge that no one else is writing their cards at this time of night.

TONIGHT'S TRIVIA

- In early English beauty parlors, women with double chins were hoisted into the air with a strap under their chin.
- Lobsters in sealed containers live longer than those with ventilation.
- In 1969 black snow fell in Sweden at Christmas.
- There are lilies growing on the Amazon that have leaves large enough to support the weight of a child.

December 14

TONIGHT'S CURE

Stay awake. Go to bed tonight with the deliberate intention of staying awake for at least one whole hour. Whatever happens you must tell yourself that you have no intention of falling asleep for that hour and will stay awake the whole time. However, the more you try and stay awake the harder it will be, and invariably people who attempt to do this are asleep within a very short time. Ironically it is a much more positive cure than setting out with the firm intention of going to sleep.

TONIGHT'S TRIVIA

• Anyone smoking twenty cigarettes a day inhales one cup full of tar a year.
• Danny Kaye made his stage debut as a watermelon seed.
• Cleopatra married two of her own brothers.
• George Washington died on December 14, 1799, the same day on which New York's World Trade Center was topped out at a height of over a quarter of a mile, in 1970.

December 15

TONIGHT'S CURE

Color change. Research has shown that color has a lot to do with sleep, and even though you may not be able to see the colors of your walls and bedclothes in the dark, they are still important and have a marked effect on you before you turn the light out. Red, for example, is a very stimulating color while the most soporific color is blue. So if you feel that your bedroom is too bright or too stimulating then you should seriously consider a color change. New walls, a new carpet, new bed covers and new sleepwear will make you feel good too. For now, however, try to visualize the color blue, absolutely nothing but pure, calm, blue—a natural sedative. Picture yourself surrounded in blue and if it helps you sleep, arrange for a change in color scheme tomorrow.

TONIGHT'S TRIVIA

• If you see a rainbow from an airplane, it will appear as a complete circle.
• Touching wood for luck stems from the early Christian belief that if you touched a piece of the cross it brought you luck.
• The first society in the world for the Prevention of Cruelty to Children was established in New York on December 15, 1874. On the same day in 1791 the U.S. Bill of Rights was ratified.
• An electric eel can produce a shock with a voltage high enough to kill a man.

December 16

TONIGHT'S CURE

Sea shore. Tonight feel your sleeplessness drain from you totally by pretending that the breath in your body is the sea. As you close your eyes and lie back it is time for low tide. Picture the tide going out, draining away from the shore, further and further. Breathe slowly and deeply feeling all the energy leaving your body with the sea, draining away so you feel heavy and cannot move a single solitary muscle. Just let yourself go with the tide. Don't worry, nothing matters anymore. Drift peacefully away towards the distant horizon and listen to the lapping waves growing fainter as they disappear into the distance.

TONIGHT'S TRIVIA

• The most powerful telescope in the world could detect a candle flame 15,500 miles away.

• *O, B, P,* and *F* are all letters that reflect the shape of the mouth as they are pronounced.

• One hundred twenty barrels of oil can be extracted from a blue whale.

• The Boston Tea Party took place on December 16, 1775, and on the same date in 1839 Abraham Lincoln met Mary Todd, his future wife.

December 17

TONIGHT'S CURE

Pushups. If you want a cure which gets you in shape while making you tired, then doing pushups each night will answer your needs. Start by lying face downward on the bedroom floor, with your forehead touching the ground. Place the palms of your hands, downward, under your shoulders. Press on the floor with your hands lifting your body into the air with your back straight, your weight supported by your arms. Extend your arms as far as they will go, and then relax them. Try to do at least twenty pushups before going to bed. Then gradually increase the number as you progress each night.

TONIGHT'S TRIVIA

• The first jeans were manufactured by one Levi Strauss, who sold them for around one dollar a pair.

• A camel's hump is pure fat.

• When you toasted a lady's health in ancient Rome you drank one glass for every letter of her name.

• Ninety-six percent of all newborn babies arrive at a time different from the one predicted by the doctor.

December 18

. . . .

TONIGHT'S CURE

Stiffness cure. Not only the elderly suffer from stiffness in the mornings; it can happen to sleepers of all ages, and anyone who frequently wakes up with a stiff shoulder each morning may experience difficulties in sleeping at night. Although we may not be conscious of it, some insomnia may be caused by the psychological fear of the morning stiffness that will confront us when we awake. Stiffness is often caused by a mattress that is too hard, even though a hard mattress is generally a good remedy for backache. To solve this problem, simply make a small soft pad to support your shoulder or whichever joint is susceptible to stiffness. You can either buy a piece of foam or else you can fold up a small blanket and place it in a pillow case. Put the pad under your shoulder and prepare for sleep. The softer the pad the better and the more relaxed you will be when you wake up in the morning free from any stiffness after a proper night's sleep.

TONIGHT'S TRIVIA

• Alphonse Durand, a Parisian music teacher, named his children Do, Re, Mi, Fa, So, La, Ti, and Do.

• In the Bible there is no mention of Jonah being swallowed by a whale.

• An electric razor uses far less energy than heating water to shave with a manual razor.

• The largest palace in the world is the Imperial Palace in Peking, which covers an area of 177.9 acres.

December 19

. . . .

TONIGHT'S CURE

Alphabetical airport. Tonight as you settle down to go to sleep, spare a thought for all those who are working and traveling through airports tonight. Turn the light out, make yourself comfortable in bed, and then imagine an airport. Start to make a list of everything in the airport, beginning with *A* for airplane, *B* for baggage, *C* for Customs, *D* for departure gate, and go on until you reach Z. Then, if you're still awake, pretend that you are on an airplane taking off at night. Picture yourself soaring into the starlit sky and drift off to sleep as you glide away through the night.

TONIGHT'S TRIVIA

- In a lifetime we breathe in enough air to fill three large airplanes.
- We shed one complete layer of skin every month.
- The earth moves around the sun eight times faster than a bullet leaves a gun.
- Jayne Mansfield had the same bust measurement as Marie Antoinette.

December 20

TONIGHT'S CURE

Festive party. The most infallible and enjoyable way of exhausting yourself completely is to give a festive party. Organize it all yourself from making the savories to eat to blowing up the balloons to organizing party games, and create an evening of nonstop entertainment for your friends. If you are very lucky you will receive a holiday gift from each one, and do make sure that everybody brings a bottle too! Then, at whatever time the party finishes, no matter how late it is, make sure you do all the washing-up and put the house straight *before* you go to bed. Nothing is worse than waking up to an untidy house and a lot of clearing up to do, and you will not sleep because it will be at the back of your mind. Instead put the house straight, then you can go to bed, exhausted, but happy and ready for sleep.

TONIGHT'S TRIVIA

- Man is the only animal that cries.
- One human hair laid on a steel bar and passed through a press would leave an imprint on the steel.
- The broad bean is the oldest known vegetable.
- Elephants are good swimmers.

December 21

TONIGHT'S CURE

White Christmas. Tonight is your chance to emulate Bing Crosby's best-selling record, *I'm Dreaming of a White Christmas,* by dreaming of a white Christmas yourself. Imagine your neighborhood covered with snow; picture the ground, the streets, the automobiles, even the people covered with thick snow. Just let the snow fall and fall and fall in your mind until everywhere and everything is completely white. Now let yourself be absorbed into this whiteness and let sleep totally envelop you.

TONIGHT'S TRIVIA

- The century plant blooms every eight years.
- If you could send a radio message to Mars it would take three and one-half minutes to get there.
- A grasshopper's legs can walk on their own when detached from the insect's body.
- As early as the time of Rameses III some Egyptian workmen went on strike for more money.

December 22

TONIGHT'S CURE

Who sent? As a means of clearing your mind, or easing a guilty conscience, lie back in bed and close your eyes. Now without using your fingers or toes, count the exact number of and note from whom you have received holiday cards. Try and visualize each card, where it is in the house, what picture is on it, and what words are inside. (It might be an idea to count exactly how many there are before you go to bed, and then calculate in your head who they are all from.)

TONIGHT'S TRIVIA

- Girls tend to sleep more soundly than boys.
- Columbus signed his name Cristobal Colon.
- The brain is not capable of feeling pain. Headaches come from the muscles and nerves around the brain.
- If you were standing on Pluto and looking at the sun, it wouldn't appear any brighter than Venus appears in the evening sky on earth.

December 23

TONIGHT'S CURE

Insomniac's holiday punch. This warming punch can be served just before you go to bed over the holiday period to help you fall into a really good, deep sleep. Mix together the following:

    2 bottles of red wine
    1 bottle of orange juice
    ½ bottle of water
    ¼ bottle of brandy.

Add allspice, nutmeg, a stick of cinnamon, and a whole orange stuck with a dozen cloves. Heat this mixture, but do not allow it to boil. When you serve the punch add sufficient liqueur brandy to ensure that the drink slips down unnoticed, save for a warming glow.

TONIGHT'S TRIVIA

• Napoleon used a bulletproof coach to travel to Waterloo.
• Cats' eyes have inner cells that reflect the light, making them glow in the dark.
• Thimbles have been in use for over three hundred years.
• President John F. Kennedy could read four newspapers straight through in twenty minutes.

December 24

TONIGHT'S CURE

Midnight Mass. Tonight's a perfect night for curing insomnia. On Christmas Eve you have an ideal reason for staying up late even if you don't have last minute holiday preparations awaiting your attention. Either visit your local church tonight for your annual Midnight Mass to celebrate the nativity, or simply join hands with your family around a log fire or tree and sing carols. Let yourself completely relax and unwind. Under no circumstances must you go to bed before midnight tonight.

TONIGHT'S TRIVIA

• The first ever television cooking demonstration showed viewers how to make an omelet.
• Horses do not have collar bones.
• Ice glaciers covered over 10 percent of the earth with debris.
• Ninety-seven percent of the water on earth is in the oceans.

December 25

TONIGHT'S CURE

Christmas cure. Tonight when you get to bed after one of the most hectic and fun-filled days of the year, cast your mind back to last Christmas Day and relive it minute by minute. Make a list of the presents you received last year and exactly who they were from. Think of all the presents you received this year. Think back to your childhood Christmases, the excitement you experienced then, and the people who made Christmas so special. Fill your mind with Christmases past and drift off to sleep in a warm glow of nostalgia.

TONIGHT'S TRIVIA

- Gabriel and Michael are the only angels mentioned in the Bible.
- In France A.M. is P.M. A.M. stands for *apres-midi* ("after noon").
- In Korea you can buy eggs on a string.
- Bubbles are round because the air pressure exerted inside them is equal in every direction.

December 26

TONIGHT'S CURE

Between *O* and *Q*. Between *O* and *Q* is that pleasant, provocative letter *P*. Repeat the letter over and over to yourself. Visualize it in your mind. Then start to list as many words as you can beginning with that letter. Play about with them on your tongue. Let a continuous stream of *P* words fall from your lips; pusillanimous, placenta, pleasure, peace, perseverance, prudence, pornographic, pastoral, placid, purity, privacy, providence, provocative, and so on until you ... pass out.

TONIGHT'S TRIVIA

- The oldest entertainment center in the world was the Colosseum in Rome which was used for over four hundred years.
- The word *love* in tennis should really be the French *l'oeuf.*
- The hairspring of a watch was originally made of a hog's hair.
- When you are struck by lightning your hair stands on end.

December 27

TONIGHT'S CURE

Loosening up. The most important preparation you can make for sleep is to loosen up all your muscles as other cures have shown. Tension builds up during the day, especially around the eyes, so you need an exercise to loosen you up completely before you go to bed. After the holidays you'll need exercise anyway. Start by standing with your legs apart and sway from one foot to the other very gently. Keep your body straight, look straight ahead, and let your arms hang completely loose. Now turn 180° to the right, with your head still facing front. Then swing 180° to the left. Allow your hips, shoulders, and arms to swing in a natural rhythm, backwards and forwards, backwards and forwards, breathing rhythmically as you swing. Continue swinging like this for five minutes and then go to bed immediately.

TONIGHT'S TRIVIA

• The name *Sierra Leone* means Lion Mountain.
• Astronauts use razors that suck in their whiskers, otherwise the bristles would float around inside the space capsule.
• Ancient Egyptians were the first to wear eternity rings.
• After the Crimean War the Russian government sold the bones of thirty-eight thousand Russian soldiers killed in action to be used as fertilizer.

December 28

· ·

TONIGHT'S CURE

Tune time. As you lie awake, allow a particular tune to come into your head, nothing too deep or heavy, but a light melody and hum it to yourself as you try to fall asleep. At the same time listen to the ticking of your bedside clock and allow the clock's rhythm to keep in time with the tune in your head. Then gradually let the clock act as a lullaby and completely take over the tune while you drift off to sleep.

TONIGHT'S TRIVIA

• In the United States, 1,400,000 eggs are laid by hens every minute.
• Cockroaches have remained unchanged on the earth for 250 million years.
• The only maroon-colored cars in Japan belong to the Imperial family.
• Czar Paul I of Russia was so conscious of his baldness that anyone who mentioned it was put to death.

December 29

· ·

TONIGHT'S CURE

Enjoy the night. Tonight you can allay your worries and fears about nighttime, you can put all the misgivings about insomnia behind you, because instead of trying not to worry about the night, that's exactly what you will be doing tonight. So turn out the light, lie back on your bed, and think about the night. Think how peaceful and tranquil it is after the rush and clamor of the day. Feel that it is your world. Look at the darkness and notice how different everything appears. Listen to the night sounds. Hear the wind, the rain, the traffic, the rustle of leaves. Smell the air, smell how fresh it is. Enjoy the fact that during these precious hours nothing else matters, your problems do not matter, there is no work to be done, and the time is yours to relax and meditate. Think of all the pleasant things in life. Take pleasure in the satisfaction of experiencing the night and the sense of one-upmanship that you have over everyone else who goes to sleep and before they know where they are it is time to start their work all over again. Enjoy these special hours alone with your thoughts until you slip gently into a deep, relaxed sleep.

TONIGHT'S TRIVIA

- The great French actress, Sarah Bernhardt, who still played youthful roles at the age of seventy, had a wooden leg.
- Over two thousand miles of yarn can be spun from one pound of cotton.
- The *chadouf* or water-raising song has been sung on the banks of the Nile for over five thousand years.
- It is against the law in New York to leave an unclothed dummy in a store window.

December 30

TONIGHT'S CURE

Happy days. Tonight, the penultimate night of the year, look back through the days and nights that have made up your year and select the high spots to enjoy again. Think of all the happy events that have taken place over the last year. Think of the new friends you have made, the new things you have bought for your house, for your family, and for yourself. Think of any improvements there have been in your job, or advances in your career. Remember happy days spent either with your family, with friends, or with the special person in your life. Think what you have gained over this year, what you now know that one year ago you were ignorant of and never dreamed would happen. Remember and relive your most enjoyable evenings, visits to the theater, TV programs, movies, and even the best books you have read. Then with all these happy memories drifting through your brain, relax and drift into a contented night's sleep.

TONIGHT'S TRIVIA

• Pure gold is soft enough to mold with your hands.
• Past kings of Spain have used the skulls of their enemies as flower pots.
• Persian carpets always contain a mistake owing to the Moslem belief that only Allah can make something that is perfect.
• The least salty sea in the world is the Baltic.

December 31

TONIGHT'S CURE

New Year's resolutions. After you have seen the New Year in tonight, which means you will not get to bed until long after midnight, look forward to the year ahead. When you are in bed, take a sheet of paper and write down all your New Year resolutions. It does not matter how small or how trivial they may seem to you, write them all down. Make resolutions—not to eat any chocolate, to cut down on cigarettes, to drink less, or to sleep more. But make certain that at the top of your list is to relax more, for this will help you sleep, to exercise more, which will make you ready for sleep, and starting from tomorrow night to work your way systematically through this book which will tell you exactly how to fall asleep. Do not stop until you have made at least thirty resolutions. Then turn out the light, lie down, and repeat the list in your mind. Tomorrow a whole New Year of living starts. Make sure that you can enjoy it by getting the sleep you need.

TONIGHT'S TRIVIA

• New Year's Eve is a popular time for predicting fortunes.
• In Sweden, molten lead is dropped into cold water and the resulting shapes are interpreted.
• Only four of Emily Dickinson's nine hundred poems were published during her lifetime.
• There is a chicken farmer in Oswego, New York, named Ted Hen. His name is also an anagram for

THE END

. . . .

DO but consider what an excellent thing sleep is: it is so inestimable a jewel that, if a tyrant would give his crown for an hour's slumber, it cannot be bought: of so beautiful a shape is it, that though a man lie with an Empress, his heart cannot beat quite till he leaves her embracements to be at rest with the other: yea, so greatly indebted are we to this kinsman of death, that we owe the better tributary, half our life to him: and there is good cause why we should do so: for sleep is the golden chain that ties health and our bodies together. Who complains of want? of wounds? of cares? of great men's oppressions? of captivity? whilst he sleepeth? Beggars in their beds take as much pleasure as kings: can we therefore surfeit of this delicate ambrosia?

—*Thomas Dekker* *1570-1632*

. . . .